OSTEOARTHRITIS DIET

COOKBOOK

For

SENIOR OVER 50

Delicious and Easy to follow Anti-inflammatory Recipes to Relieve Arthritis Pain, Enhance Joint Health and Boost Mobility

ANGELA R. STATEN

TABLE OF CONTENTS

ABOUT THE AUTHOR

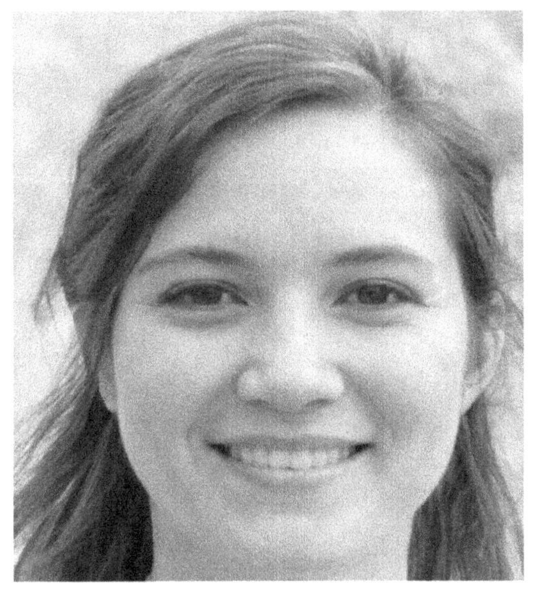

My name is Angela Rachel Staten, and I'm a medical professional and qualified nutritionist who is totally committed to using food as medicine.

Although it may sound generic, I have personally witnessed the profound impact that a healthy diet can have on people's lives.

I am a case study in action.

Whether you have Arthritis or are facing another health issue, my intention is not to give you a ton of confusing guidelines.

Rather, I wish to provide you with the means to effect long-term change.

One of the greatest methods to achieve this is by following a healthy diet, which focuses on eating tasty but simple foods that will fuel your body and provide you with the strongest defense against illness.

You will find in this book:

Clear explanations of the nutritional value of food and how it affects leading a healthy lifestyle.

scrumptious meals that genuinely inspire a desire for healthy eating.

Some pointers for incorporating this diet into your busy lifestyle.

Consider myself your companion in this. One delectable, nutritious meal at a time, I'm here to help you on your path to feeling better.

Let's get started.

INTRODUCTION

Are you over 50 and feeling the occasional stiffness or twinge in your joints? Perhaps the daily walks you used to enjoy now come with a bit more discomfort. If you've been diagnosed with osteoarthritis, you're certainly not alone.

This book is your personalized guide to a delicious and effective journey towards better joint health.

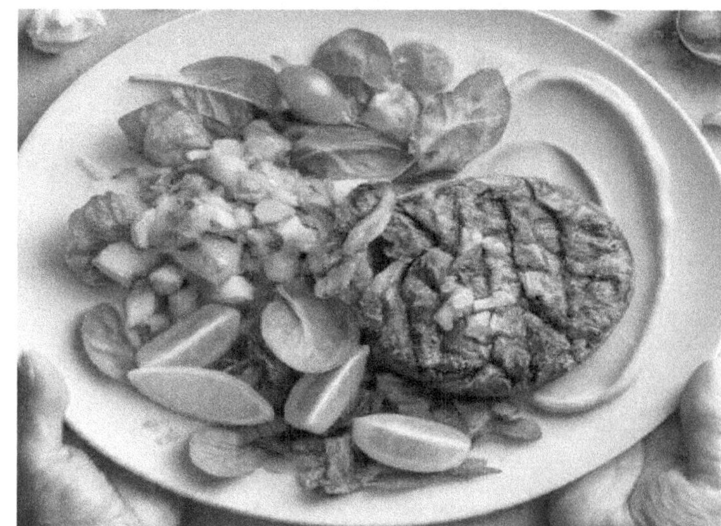

We understand the frustration and limitations that osteoarthritis can bring, and we're here to empower you with knowledge and practical tools.

Within these pages, you'll discover the surprising connection between what you eat and the health of your joints.

We'll explore the science behind anti-inflammatory foods and how they can significantly reduce pain and stiffness.

You'll learn about essential nutrients for strong bones and muscles, all while fueling your body with delicious and satisfying recipes.

This isn't just a cookbook; it's a comprehensive resource designed specifically for seniors over 50.

We'll provide easy-to-follow advice on mindful eating, grocery shopping with osteoarthritis in mind, and adapting your favorite recipes for a joint-friendly twist. Whether you're a seasoned cook or just starting to explore the kitchen, we've got you covered.

More importantly, we'll be your partner on this journey. We understand the unique challenges that seniors face, and we'll offer guidance and support every step of the way.

So, turn the page, grab your apron, and get ready to experience the transformative power of food for a healthier, more vibrant you!

Take Note:

CHAPTER 1

Introduction to Osteoarthritis

What is osteoarthritis?

Osteoarthritis (OA) might sound complex, but it's actually a common condition that affects many seniors over 50.

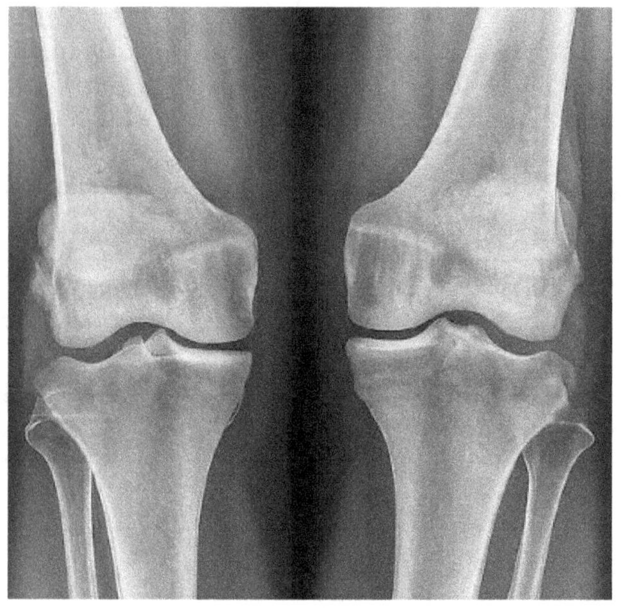

Think of your joints as the hinges in your body, allowing you to move with ease. In osteoarthritis, the smooth cartilage that cushions these joints starts to wear down over time. This can cause:

Pain: You might feel an ache or stiffness in your joints, especially after activity or at the end of the day.

Stiffness: Your joints may feel a little tight or stuck, particularly in the mornings or after resting for a while.

Reduced Flexibility: Simple movements like bending down or reaching for something overhead might become a bit more challenging.

Here's a breakdown of what happens in osteoarthritis:

Cartilage Cushioning: Imagine the cartilage in your joints like the pads in your sneakers. They absorb shock and keep the bones from rubbing together painfully.

Breakdown and Wear: Over time, due to various factors like age, injury, or overuse, this cartilage can wear down and become thin or even break down completely.

Bone Rubbing: When the cartilage wears away, the underlying bones start to rub together. This can cause inflammation, pain, and swelling in the joint.

While osteoarthritis can't be reversed, there's a lot you can do to manage your symptoms and feel better.

This book will be your guide, focusing on how a healthy diet packed with the right nutrients can significantly reduce inflammation and support your joint health.

So let's explore.

Symptoms and diagnosis

Osteoarthritis can affect any joint in your body, but it most commonly targets areas that bear weight, such as:

- Knees
- Hips
- Hands
- Spine (lower back)
- Big toes

The symptoms of osteoarthritis often develop gradually over time and can vary from person to person.

Here's what to look out for:

Joint Pain: This is the most common symptom, often described as an aching or stiffness that worsens with activity, particularly weight-bearing exercises like walking or climbing stairs.

The pain might also be more pronounced at the end of the day or after prolonged sitting.

Joint Stiffness: You may experience stiffness in your joints, especially upon waking up or after periods of inactivity. This stiffness usually improves with gentle movement.

Reduced Range of Motion: Osteoarthritis can limit the flexibility of your joints, making it more difficult to perform certain movements. For example, reaching for something high on a shelf or bending down to tie your shoes might become more challenging.

Joint Swelling: Sometimes, the affected joint may become swollen, red, or tender to the touch. This is due to inflammation caused by the breakdown of cartilage.

Grating or Popping Sounds: You might hear or feel a sensation of grinding, creaking, or popping when you move your joints. This is caused by the bones rubbing together in the absence of smooth cartilage cushioning.

Diagnosis of Osteoarthritis

There's no single test to diagnose osteoarthritis.

Your doctor will likely ask about your medical history, symptoms, and lifestyle habits.

They may also perform a physical examination to assess your range of motion, joint tenderness, and swelling.

In some cases, your doctor may recommend imaging tests like X-rays to visualize the bones and assess the extent of cartilage damage.

However, X-rays don't directly show cartilage, so other imaging techniques like MRIs might be used in specific situations.

It's important to note that these symptoms can sometimes mimic other conditions.

If you're experiencing any of these issues, it's crucial to consult your doctor for a proper diagnosis and discuss the best course of treatment for you.

Risk factors and common concerns for seniors.

Osteoarthritis is a prevalent condition among seniors over 50, but certain factors can increase your risk of developing it.

Below is a summary of some typical risk factors:

Age: As we age, the cartilage in our joints naturally breaks down, making us more susceptible to osteoarthritis.

Previous Injuries: Joint injuries, even those sustained years ago, can damage cartilage and increase the risk of osteoarthritis later in life.

Overweight and Obesity: Excess body weight puts extra stress on weight-bearing joints like knees and hips, accelerating cartilage wear and tear.

Genetics: Some people have a genetic predisposition towards developing osteoarthritis.

Repetitive Stress: Jobs or hobbies that involve repetitive movements of specific joints can increase the risk of osteoarthritis in those areas.

Common Concerns for Seniors with Osteoarthritis

We understand that living with osteoarthritis can raise a number of concerns.

Here are some of the most common ones and some reassuring thoughts:

Loss of Independence: You might worry that your mobility will be limited, hindering your ability to live independently. This book will equip you with strategies to manage your condition and maintain an active lifestyle.

Pain Management: Pain can be a significant concern, but we'll explore dietary approaches that can help reduce inflammation and ease discomfort.

Staying Active: Physical activity is crucial for overall health and joint health. We'll provide guidance on low-impact exercises and lifestyle modifications that can keep you moving without worsening your symptoms.

Maintaining a Healthy Weight: Weight management plays a vital role in managing osteoarthritis. We'll offer delicious recipes and tips for portion control to help you achieve and maintain a healthy weight.

Take Note:

CHAPTER 2

The Anti-Inflammatory Diet Connection

How inflammation impacts osteoarthritis

Osteoarthritis is often described as a "wear and tear" condition, but there's more to the story. Inflammation plays a crucial role in its development and progression. Here's a closer look at this link and how dietary choices can make a significant difference:

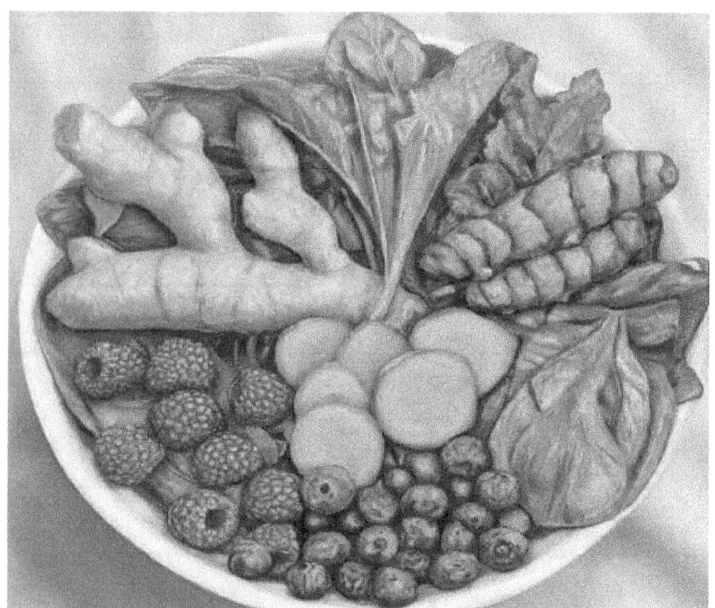

The Inflammation Connection:

Think of your joints as a well-oiled machine. The smooth cartilage acts as a cushion, ensuring frictionless movement.

In osteoarthritis, this cartilage starts to break down. However, the body's response goes beyond just repairing the damage.

The breakdown of cartilage triggers an inflammatory response, releasing chemicals called cytokines.

Cytokines and Cartilage Damage:

These cytokines act like messengers, sending signals to the surrounding tissues. Unfortunately, in the case of osteoarthritis, these signals can be destructive.

They stimulate the production of enzymes that further break down cartilage, creating a vicious cycle of inflammation and damage.

The Domino Effect of Inflammation:

Chronic inflammation can also lead to:

Increased pain and stiffness: Inflammation sensitizes the nerves around the joint, amplifying pain perception and causing stiffness.

Swelling and tenderness: Inflammation triggers fluid buildup in the joint, leading to swelling and tenderness.

Bone spur formation: In some cases, chronic inflammation can stimulate the growth of bony projections (osteophytes) around the joint, further restricting movement.

Food as your savior:

The good news is that you can influence this inflammatory process through your diet! Certain foods act as natural anti-inflammatory agents, while others can contribute to inflammation. By incorporating anti-inflammatory foods into your diet and limiting those that promote inflammation, you can significantly reduce the burden on your joints and manage your osteoarthritis symptoms more effectively.

This book will be your guide to navigating the world of anti-inflammatory foods. We'll explore the science behind these powerful ingredients and provide you with delicious recipes that are not only good for your taste buds but also beneficial for your joints. Remember, with the right dietary choices, you can empower your body to fight inflammation and experience better joint health.

The role of diet in reducing inflammation and managing symptoms.

While there's no magic bullet to cure osteoarthritis, the power of food can significantly reduce inflammation and manage your symptoms, allowing you to live a more active and fulfilling life.

Here's how a well-planned, anti-inflammatory diet can be your weapon in combating osteoarthritis:

Quenching the Inflammatory Fire:

As we discussed earlier, inflammation plays a key role in the progression of osteoarthritis. Certain foods act as pro-inflammatory agents, while others have potent anti-inflammatory properties.

By adding these anti-inflammatory ingredients into your diet, you can help:

Reduce Cytokine Production: Anti-inflammatory foods can dampen the production of inflammatory cytokines, putting the brakes on cartilage breakdown.

Minimize Pain and Stiffness: By reducing inflammation, you can experience a significant decrease in pain and stiffness in your joints, improving your overall well-being.

Support Joint Repair: Some dietary components can even promote the repair and regeneration of healthy joint tissues.

Dietary Stars for Osteoarthritis Management

Here are some key dietary heroes that will be featured throughout this book:

Fruits and Vegetables: They're packed with antioxidants that combat inflammation. Deeply colored fruits and vegetables, like berries, leafy greens, and bell peppers, are particularly rich in these beneficial compounds.

Omega-3 Fatty Acids: Found in fatty fish like salmon, tuna, and sardines, omega-3s are renowned for their anti-inflammatory properties. They can help reduce joint pain and stiffness, making movement easier.

Healthy Fats: Not all fats are created equal! Opt for healthy fats like those found in olive oil, avocados, and nuts. These fats possess anti-inflammatory properties and contribute to a feeling of satiety, aiding in weight management, which further benefits your joints.

Whole Grains: Whole grains are a source of complex carbohydrates and fiber, which can help regulate blood sugar levels and promote gut health. Both factors can contribute to reducing inflammation throughout the body.

Take Note:

CHAPTER 3

Dietary Considerations for Seniors with Osteoarthritis

Nutritional needs of seniors over 50

As we enter our golden years, our nutritional needs shift slightly. Our metabolism may slow down, and our bodies may require different nutrients to function optimally.

This section will talk about the specific nutritional needs of seniors over 50, particularly those managing osteoarthritis, to ensure you're getting the essential building blocks for good health and joint support.

Essential Macronutrients:

Protein: Protein is crucial for building and maintaining muscle mass, which helps support joint health and stability. Seniors are at an increased risk of muscle loss (sarcopenia), so ensuring adequate protein intake becomes even more important. Lean protein sources like chicken, fish, beans, and lentils will be highlighted throughout this book.

Carbohydrates: While refined carbohydrates like white bread and pastries can contribute to inflammation, complex carbohydrates from whole grains are essential for providing sustained energy. These complex carbohydrates are also a good source of fiber, which promotes gut health and may indirectly reduce inflammation.

Healthy Fats: Don't shy away from healthy fats! Including healthy fats like those found in olive oil, avocados, and nuts in your diet is vital. These fats not only provide satiety and support weight management but also possess anti-inflammatory properties beneficial for joint health.

Micronutrients and Bone Health:

Calcium and Vitamin D: These powerhouse nutrients work together to maintain strong bones, which is particularly important for preventing fractures as we age. This book will explore various dietary sources of calcium and vitamin D, as well as the importance of consulting your doctor about potential supplementation if needed.

Vitamin K: Emerging research suggests Vitamin K may play a role in bone health and blood clotting. While more research is ongoing, we'll discuss incorporating Vitamin K-rich foods like leafy green vegetables into your diet.

Staying Hydrated:

Water is Essential: Dehydration can worsen joint stiffness and pain. Aiming for eight glasses of water daily is crucial for overall health and joint lubrication. We'll provide tips on increasing your water intake and incorporating hydrating fruits and vegetables into your diet.

Individualized Needs:

It's important to remember that these are general guidelines. Seniors may have other health conditions co-existing with osteoarthritis, which might necessitate specific dietary adjustments. We'll emphasize the importance of consulting a doctor or registered dietitian for personalized advice tailored to your unique needs.

- Importance of maintaining a healthy weight.
- Adapting the diet for common coexisting conditions
- Osteoarthritis often joins hands with other health concerns in seniors over 50.

While the core principles of an anti-inflammatory diet remain the foundation, there might be a need for some adjustments based on co-existing conditions. This section will offer guidance on adapting your diet to manage these conditions alongside osteoarthritis:

High Blood Pressure: Focus on Low-Sodium Options: Limit processed foods, canned goods, and added table salt. Opt for fresh herbs and spices to add flavor to your dishes.

Embrace Fruits and Vegetables: These are naturally low in sodium and rich in potassium, a mineral that helps regulate blood pressure.

Moderate Protein Intake: While protein is essential, excessive intake can put a strain on the kidneys. Choose lean protein sources and focus on portion control.

High Cholesterol: Limit Saturated and Trans Fats: These fats can elevate LDL ("bad") cholesterol levels. Minimize red meat, processed meats, and fried foods.

Embrace Healthy Fats: Include healthy fats like those found in olive oil, avocados, and fatty fish in your diet. These fats promote HDL ("good") cholesterol and have anti-inflammatory properties.

Fiber is Your Friend: Soluble fiber in oats, beans, and certain fruits can help trap cholesterol and eliminate it from the body.

Diabetes: Focus on Blood Sugar Control: Choose whole grains, fruits with a lower glycemic index (GI), and lean protein sources to maintain stable blood sugar levels.

Mind Your Portion Sizes: Manage portion control to avoid blood sugar spikes.

Limit Refined Carbohydrates: Sugary drinks, white bread, and pastries can significantly impact blood sugar. Opt for complex carbohydrates with a lower GI.

key point to note:

Consult Your Doctor: It's crucial to discuss any dietary modifications with your doctor or registered dietitian to ensure they align with your specific treatment plan for co-existing conditions.

Individualized Approach: The adjustments listed here are general recommendations. Your doctor will guide you based on the severity of your co-existing conditions and medication use.

Take Note:

CHAPTER 4

Essential Anti-Inflammatory Foods

The following are essential anti-inflammatory foods

Category	Foods
Fruits	Acai, Apples, Avocado, Blackberries, Blueberries, Cantaloupe, Cherries, Cranberries, Grapefruit, Grapes, Lemon, Mango, Oranges, Papaya, Passionfruit, Pears, Pineapple, Plums, Raspberries, Star fruit, Tangerines, Tomatoes, Watermelon
Vegetables	Artichoke, Asparagus, Beets, Bok choy, Broccoli, Brussels sprouts, Cabbage (red and green), Carrots, Celery, Collard greens, Garlic, Jicama, Kale, Mushrooms, Onions, Bell peppers (orange, red, yellow), Parsley, Pumpkin, Spaghetti squash, Spinach, Sweet potato, Turnips, Turnip greens, Yellow bell peppers
Grains	Amaranth, Barley, Brown rice, Buckwheat, Millet, Oats (steel cut or whole), Quinoa, Wheat germ
Protein Sources	Almonds, Anchovies, Black beans, Chickpeas (garbanzo beans), Chia seeds, Cod, Flaxseed, Hazelnuts, Hemp seeds, Herring, Kidney beans, Lentils, Lima beans, Mackerel, Peanuts, Peas, Salmon, Sardines, Soybeans (including tofu), Sunflower seeds, Tuna, Walnuts

Other Anti-inflammatory Power Players

Avocado oil: Healthy fat with anti-inflammatory properties, suitable for cooking or drizzling on salads and vegetables.

Cayenne pepper: Spice containing capsaicin, a compound with potential anti-inflammatory properties.

Cinnamon: Spice with some anti-inflammatory properties, also beneficial for blood sugar control.

Cumin: Spice with potential anti-inflammatory effects.

Dark chocolate (high cocoa content, in moderation): Contains flavanols, which have some anti-inflammatory effects. But because it contains sugar, it's crucial to eat it in moderation.

Flaxseed oil: Source of ALA, an omega-3 fatty acid with potential anti-inflammatory effects.

Ginger: Spice with well-documented anti-inflammatory properties.

Green tea: Source of antioxidants with potential anti-inflammatory benefits.

Olive oil: Healthy fat with anti-inflammatory properties, suitable for cooking or drizzling on salads and vegetables.

Turmeric: Spice containing curcumin, a compound with potent anti-inflammatory properties.

Walnut oil: Source of healthy fats with some potential anti-inflammatory effects

Complete Anti-Inflammatory Food List for Osteoarthritis

Category	Anti-Inflammatory Foods
Fruits	Acai, Apples, Avocado, Blackberries, Blueberries, Cantaloupe, Cherries, Cranberries, Grapefruit, Grapes, Lemon, Mango, Oranges, Papaya, Passionfruit, Pears, Pineapple (in moderation), Plums, Raspberries, Star fruit, Tangerines, Tomatoes, Watermelon (in moderation)
Vegetables	Artichoke, Asparagus, Beets, Bok choy, Broccoli, Brussels sprouts, Cabbage (red and green), Carrots, Celery, Collard greens, Garlic, Jicama, Kale, Mushrooms, Onions, Bell peppers (orange, red, yellow), Parsley, Pumpkin, Spaghetti squash, Spinach, Sweet potato, Turnips, Turnip greens, Yellow bell peppers
Grains	Amaranth, Barley, Brown rice, Buckwheat, Millet, Oats (steel-cut or whole), Quinoa, Wheat germ
Protein Sources	Almonds, Anchovies, Black beans, Chickpeas, Chia seeds, Cod, Flaxseed, Hazelnuts, Hemp seeds, Herring, Kidney beans, Lentils, Lima beans, Mackerel, Peanuts (allergy caution), Peas, Salmon, Sardines, Soybeans (including tofu), Sunflower seeds, Tuna, Walnuts

| Other | Avocado oil, Cayenne pepper, Cinnamon, Cumin, Dark chocolate (high cocoa, in moderation), Flaxseed oil, Ginger, Green tea, Olive oil, Turmeric, Walnut oil |

Foods to Avoid for Inflammation

Category	Foods to Limit or Avoid
Processed Foods	Commercially baked goods (cookies, cakes, pastries), packaged snacks (chips, crackers), sugary drinks (soda, juice), processed meats (deli meats, hot dogs), frozen dinners and pre-made meals.
Refined Carbohydrates	White bread and pasta, white rice, sugary cereals.
Unhealthy Fats	Saturated fats (fatty meats, full-fat dairy), trans fats (fried foods, some baked goods, some margarines).
Other	Excessive alcohol, refined vegetable oils (corn oil, soybean oil), added sugars (candy, desserts, sugary drinks).

Take Note:

CHAPTER 5

Hydration and Joint Health

Importance of staying hydrated for joints

Taking care of your joints is crucial, especially as we age. They're the hinges that allow us to move freely, stay active, and enjoy life to the fullest. But did you know that one of the simplest and most effective ways to keep your joints healthy is by staying hydrated?

Here's why water is your secret weapon for healthy joints:

Lubrication: Your joints are intricate structures that contain cartilage, a rubbery tissue that cushions the bones and allows for smooth movement. Cartilage is about 80% water! When you're dehydrated, the cartilage loses its ability to absorb shock and becomes more susceptible to wear and tear. Think of it like a car with deflated tires – it's bumpier and more prone to damage.

Nutrient Delivery: Just like all other parts of your body, your joints need proper nourishment. Water transports vital nutrients, like calcium and glucosamine, to the cartilage cells, keeping them healthy and strong.

Waste Removal: During physical activity, your joints produce waste products. Proper hydration helps flush out these toxins, preventing inflammation and pain.

Shock Absorber: The synovial fluid surrounding your joints acts like a shock absorber, cushioning the bones and reducing friction. This fluid is primarily composed of water. Dehydration can decrease the amount of synovial fluid, leading to increased stress on the joints and potential pain.

Signs of Dehydration and Joint Health

- Feeling thirsty is a late sign of dehydration. Here are some earlier signs to watch out for:
- Feeling tired or sluggish
- Headaches
- Dry mouth
- Decreased urination (dark yellow urine)

- Stiffness in the joints

Note: If you experience these symptoms, especially after physical activity, it's a good indication that you need to increase your water intake.

Tips for increasing water intake in seniors.

Staying hydrated is crucial for everyone, but it becomes especially important for seniors as their bodies become less efficient at managing fluids. Dehydration can lead to a variety of health problems, including constipation, urinary tract infections, and even dizziness. The good news is there are simple strategies seniors can incorporate into their daily routine to ensure they're getting enough water.

Make it Easy and Accessible:

Carry a reusable water bottle: Invest in a comfortable, insulated water bottle with a straw or easy-to-open lid. Keep it filled and readily available throughout the day, especially during outings or walks.

Set Reminders: Utilize alarms on phones or watches or place sticky notes around the house as visual cues to sip on water throughout the day.

Pair water with activities: Develop a habit of drinking a glass of water before meals, with medications, upon waking up, and before going to bed.

Make it Appealing:

Infuse your water: Add slices of lemon, cucumber, berries, or mint leaves for a touch of natural flavor and a visual invitation to drink.

Explore different temperatures: Some seniors prefer chilled water, while others enjoy it lukewarm with a squeeze of lemon. Experiment to find what's most appealing.

Consider sparkling water: Opt for sugar-free sparkling water with a splash of fruit juice for a refreshing alternative.

Additional Tips:

Focus on small, frequent sips: Instead of aiming for a large volume at once, aim for smaller, more frequent sips throughout the day.

Choose water-rich foods: Incorporate plenty of fruits and vegetables with high water content into your diet, such as watermelon, cantaloupe, celery, oranges, and tomatoes. Your daily fluid intake is influenced by these foods.

Monitor urine color: Good hydration can be detected by pale yellow urine.

Darker yellow urine suggests dehydration, prompting you to increase your water intake.

Consult with your doctor: If you have any underlying health conditions that affect fluid intake or medication causing dryness, discuss water intake strategies with your doctor.

Involve family and caregivers: Family members and caregivers can play a supportive role by reminding seniors to drink water and making sure their water bottle is always refilled and accessible.

Take Note:

CHAPTER 6

BREAKFAST RECIPES

BERRY BLAST SMOOTHIE

Yields: 1 Serving | **Prep Time**: 5 minutes | **Cook Time**: No Cook

INGREDIENTS

- 1 cup frozen blueberries
- ½ cup frozen raspberries
- ½ cup frozen blackberries
- ½ cup unsweetened almond milk (or other preferred milk)
- 1 tablespoon ground flaxseed
- 1 tablespoon honey (optional)

INSTRUCTIONS

1. Wash all fruits thoroughly, even if frozen.
2. Dry them off using a fresh paper towel.
3. Add all ingredients to a blender.
4. Blend on high speed until smooth and creamy. You may need to stop and scrape down the sides a couple of times for even blending.
5. If using honey for additional sweetness, add it to taste after blending and blend again briefly.
6. Pour into a glass and enjoy!

- Feel free to adjust the amount of fruit based on your taste preference.

- To add even more protein, you can mix in a scoop of protein powder.

- If the smoothie is too thick, add a little more milk, one tablespoon at a time, until it reaches your desired consistency.

- Frozen fruits add thickness to the smoothie, but you can also use fresh fruits and add some ice cubes for a chilled drink.

NUTRITIONAL FACTS

Calories: 200-250 (depending on the type of milk used and added honey)

Protein: 4 grams

Fiber: 6 grams

Vitamin C: Excellent source

Manganese: Excellent source

Antioxidants: High

TROPICAL POWER BOWL

Yields: 1 Serving | **Prep Time:** 5 minutes| **Cook Time:** No Cook

INGREDIENTS

- ½ cup chopped mango
- ½ cup chopped papaya
- ¼ cup frozen acai berries
- ½ cup plain Greek yogurt
- 1 tablespoon chia seeds
- Toppings (optional): Sliced almonds, shredded coconut, granola

INSTRUCTIONS

1. Wash and chop the mango and papaya.
2. In a bowl, combine the chopped fruits, acai berries, Greek yogurt, and chia seeds.
3. Top with your favorite toppings like sliced almonds, shredded coconut, or granola (optional).

- If you don't have fresh acai berries, you can use acai powder (½ - 1 teaspoon) mixed with a little water to create a paste before adding it to the bowl.
- Frozen chopped mango and papaya can be used instead of fresh ones.
- This recipe is easily customizable. You can substitute other fruits you enjoy like pineapple, kiwi, or berries.

NUTRITIONAL FACTS

Calories: 300-350 (depending on toppings)

Protein: 15 grams (from Greek yogurt)

Fiber: 6 grams

Vitamin C: Excellent source (from mango and papaya)

Antioxidants: High

TURMERIC TOFU SCRAMBLE

Yields: 1 Serving | **Prep Time:** 10 minutes | **Cook Time:** 10 minutes

INGREDIENTS

- 4 ounces firm tofu, crumbled
- ½ teaspoon turmeric powder
- ¼ teaspoon paprika
- ¼ teaspoon ground black pepper
- ¼ teaspoon garlic powder
- ½ red bell pepper, chopped
- ¼ yellow bell pepper, chopped
- ¼ cup chopped onion
- 1 tablespoon olive oil
- ¼ cup chopped fresh parsley (optional)
- Iodized sea salt to taste

INSTRUCTIONS

1. Drain and press the tofu. You can do this by wrapping it in a clean kitchen towel and placing a heavy object on top for 10-15 minutes.
2. While the tofu is pressing, heat the olive oil in a skillet over medium heat.
3. Add the chopped onion and bell peppers to the pan and cook for 5 minutes, or until softened.
4. Crumble the pressed tofu into the pan with the vegetables.
5. Add the turmeric powder, paprika, black pepper, and garlic powder. Stir to coat the tofu evenly.
6. Cook for another 5-7 minutes, or until the tofu is golden brown and heated through.
7. Season with iodized sea salt to taste.
8. Garnish with chopped fresh parsley (optional) and serve immediately.

TIPS

- To make the tofu scramble even more flavorful, you can add a tablespoon of nutritional yeast or a splash of soy sauce.
- Cooking for Two: Simply double all ingredient quantities for a two-serving recipe.
- Storage: Smoothies are best enjoyed fresh. Leftovers from the Tropical Power Bowl or Turmeric Tofu Scramble can be stored in an airtight container in the refrigerator for up to 2 days.
- Gently reheat in a skillet or microwave just before serving.

NUTRITIONAL FACTS

Calories: 300-350

Protein: 20 grams

Fiber: 2 grams

Iron: Good source

Calcium: Good source (from fortified tofu)

SWEET POTATO PANCAKES

Yields: 2-3 servings | **Prep Time:** 10 minutes | **Cook Time:** 15 minutes

INGREDIENTS

- 1 medium sweet potato (about 1 cup mashed)
- ½ cup rolled oats
- 1 egg, beaten
- 1 teaspoon ground cinnamon
- ¼ teaspoon ground ginger (optional, anti-inflammatory)
- ¼ teaspoon nutmeg (optional)
- ¼ teaspoon iodized sea salt
- 1 tablespoon olive oil

INSTRUCTIONS

1. Wash the sweet potato and prick it with a fork a few times. Microwave on high for 5-7 minutes, or until tender. You can also bake it in the oven at 400°F (200°C) for about 45 minutes, or until soft.
2. Once cooked, let the sweet potato cool slightly. Peel it and mash it with a fork or potato masher until smooth.
3. In a large bowl, combine the mashed sweet potato, rolled oats, beaten egg, cinnamon, ginger (if using), nutmeg (if using), and sea salt. Till everything is well incorporated, thoroughly mixed.
4. Heat the olive oil in a non-stick skillet over medium heat.
5. Scoop about ¼ cup of the batter for each pancake onto the hot skillet.
6. Cook for 3-4 minutes per side, or until golden brown and cooked through. You can gently press down on the pancakes with a spatula while cooking to help them cook evenly.
7. Serve warm with your favorite toppings like fresh berries, chopped nuts, or a drizzle of maple syrup (use sparingly).

- For a thicker batter, add a little more rolled oats, one tablespoon at a time, until you reach the desired consistency.
- Leftover pancakes can be stored in an airtight container in the refrigerator for up to 2 days. Gently reheat in a skillet or microwave just before serving.

NUTRITIONAL FACTS

Calories: 150-200

Protein: 4 grams

Fiber: 3 grams

Vitamin A: Excellent source (from sweet potato)

Manganese: Good source

SALMON AND AVOCADO TOAST

Yields: 1 Serving | **Prep Time:** 5 minutes | **Cook Time:** No Cook

INGREDIENTS

- 1 slice whole wheat bread, toasted
- 2-3 ounces cooked salmon (grilled, baked, or poached)
- ½ ripe avocado, sliced
- Lemon juice (optional)
- Freshly ground black pepper
- Iodized sea salt to taste

INSTRUCTIONS

1. Toast a slice of whole wheat bread to your desired level of doneness.
2. Flake the cooked salmon and arrange it on the toasted bread.
3. Top with sliced avocado. You can drizzle a little lemon juice on the avocado to prevent browning (optional).
4. Season with freshly ground black pepper and iodized sea salt to taste.

- Feel free to add other toppings to your toast like sliced tomatoes, cucumbers, or a sprinkle of chopped chives.
- Leftover cooked salmon can be used for this recipe.
- You can also use canned salmon, but be sure to choose a variety packed in water instead of oil.

NUTRITIONAL FACTS

Calories: 300-350

Protein: 20 grams (from salmon)

Healthy fats: Excellent source (from salmon and avocado)

Vitamin D: Excellent source (from salmon)

SPICED OATMEAL WITH BERRIES

Yields: 1 Serving | **Prep Time**: 5 minutes | **Cook Time**: 10 minutes

INGREDIENTS

- ½ cup rolled oats
- One cup of unsweetened almond milk, or any other plant-based milk of choice
- ¼ cup water
- ½ teaspoon ground cinnamon
- ¼ teaspoon ground ginger (optional, anti-inflammatory)
- ¼ teaspoon ground nutmeg (optional)
- Pinch of iodized sea salt
- ¼ cup fresh or frozen berries
- 1 tablespoon chopped almonds (optional)

INSTRUCTIONS

1. In a saucepan, combine the rolled oats, almond milk, water, cinnamon, ginger (if using), nutmeg (if using), and sea salt.

2. Bring to a boil over medium heat.

3. Reduce heat to low and simmer for 5-7 minutes, or until the oats are cooked through and the oatmeal reaches your desired consistency. Stir occasionally to prevent sticking.

4. Remove from heat and stir in the berries.

5. Top with chopped almonds (optional) and serve warm.

- For a sweeter oatmeal, you can add a teaspoon of honey or maple syrup after cooking. However, use these sparingly as they contain added sugars.
- You can customize this recipe with other toppings like sliced banana, chopped nuts, or a sprinkle of chia seeds.
- Oatmeal leftovers keep well in the refrigerator for up to two days when kept in an airtight container.
- Gently reheat in a skillet or microwave ahead of serving.

NUTRITIONAL FACTS

Calories: 250-300

Protein: 4 grams

Fiber: 4 grams

Manganese: Good source

CHERRY TOMATO AND SPINACH FRITTATA

Yields: 1-2 servings | **Prep Time:** 10 minutes | **Cook Time:** 20-25 minutes

INGREDIENTS

- 3 large eggs
- ¼ cup unsweetened almond milk (or other preferred plantbased milk)
- ½ cup chopped fresh spinach
- ½ cup halved cherry tomatoes
- ¼ teaspoon dried oregano (optional)
- ¼ teaspoon ground black pepper
- Iodized sea salt to taste
- 1 tablespoon olive oil

INSTRUCTIONS

1. Preheat your oven to 375°F (190°C). Lightly grease a small oven-safe skillet or pie dish.
2. In a large bowl, whisk together the eggs and almond milk. Season with black pepper and a pinch of sea salt.
3. Stir in the chopped spinach, halved cherry tomatoes, and dried oregano (if using).
4. Heat the olive oil in your preheated skillet over medium heat. Once heated, add the egg mixture.
5. Tilt the pan occasionally to allow the uncooked egg to move towards the edges.
6. As the bottom begins to set, reduce heat to low and cook for 10-12 minutes, or until the edges are set but the center is still slightly runny.
7. Transfer the skillet to the preheated oven and bake for another 5-7 minutes, or until the center is cooked through.
8. Take out of the oven and allow it to cool down a little bit before slicing and serving.

- Feel free to add other chopped vegetables to your frittata like chopped bell peppers, mushrooms, or onions.
- Leftover frittata can be stored in an airtight container in the refrigerator for up to 3 days.
- Gently reheat in a skillet or microwave ahead of serving.
- You can also enjoy frittata cold for a refreshing breakfast or lunch option.

NUTRITIONAL FACTS

Calories: 200-250

Protein: 12 grams

Vitamin K: Excellent source (from spinach)

Choline: Good source (from eggs)

POWER GREENS SMOOTHIE

Yields: 1 Serving | **Prep Time:** 5 minutes | **Cook Time:** No Cook

INGREDIENTS

- 1 cup chopped kale
- ½ cup chopped spinach
- ½ pear, chopped
- ½ inch fresh ginger, peeled and chopped (anti-inflammatory)
- One cup of unsweetened almond milk, or any other plant-based milk of choice
- ½ cup water (optional, adjust for desired consistency)

INSTRUCTIONS

1. Wash all fruits and vegetables thoroughly.
2. Add all ingredients to a blender.
3. Blend on high speed until smooth and creamy. You may need to stop and scrape down the sides a couple of times for even blending.
4. Add a little more water or milk, one tablespoon at a time, if the smoothie is too thick.
5. Pour into a glass and enjoy!

TIPS

- Use one-half teaspoon of ground ginger in place of fresh ginger.

- You can substitute the pear with another fruit you enjoy like banana, apple, or berries.

- For an extra protein boost, add a scoop of protein powder to your smoothie.

NUTRITIONAL FACTS

Calories: 200-250

Vitamin C: Excellent source (from kale and spinach)

Vitamin K: Excellent source (from kale)

Manganese: Excellent source

OVERNIGHT OATS WITH NUTS AND SEEDS

Yields: 1 Serving | **Prep Time:** 5 minutes | **Cook Time:** No Cook

INGREDIENTS

- ½ cup rolled oats
- ½ cup unsweetened Greek yogurt
- ¼ cup unsweetened almond milk (or other preferred milk)
- ¼ cup chopped walnuts
- 1 tablespoon sliced almonds
- 1 tablespoon chia seeds
- ¼ teaspoon ground cinnamon
- Pinch of iodized sea salt

INSTRUCTIONS

1. In a small jar or container, combine the rolled oats, Greek yogurt, almond milk, chopped walnuts, sliced almonds, chia seeds, ground cinnamon, and a pinch of sea salt.
2. Stir well to combine and make sure the oats are coated evenly.
3. Cover the jar or container tightly and refrigerate overnight for at least 8 hours, or up to 2 nights.
4. In the morning, stir the oatmeal again and enjoy it cold.

- Feel free to customize this recipe with other chopped nuts and seeds like pecans, sunflower seeds, or pumpkin seeds.
- You can also add a drizzle of honey or maple syrup for a touch of sweetness in the morning. However, use these sparingly as they contain added sugars.
- Overnight oats can be layered with fresh fruit slices like berries or chopped mango for added flavor and texture

NUTRITIONAL FACTS

Calories: 300-350

Protein: 15 grams (from Greek yogurt)

Fiber: 6 grams

Healthy fats: Good source (from nuts and seeds)

Calcium: Good source (from Greek yogurt)

Vitamin E: Good source (from nuts and seeds)

QUINOA PANCAKES WITH BERRIES

Yields: 2-3 servings | **Prep Time:** 10 minutes | **Cook Time:** 15 minutes

INGREDIENTS

- ½ cup cooked quinoa
- ½ cup rolled oats
- One cup of almond milk, unsweetened, or your favorite plant based milk.
- 1 egg, beaten
- 1 tablespoon ground flaxseed (mixed with 3 tablespoons water and let sit for 5 minutes, creates a flax "egg")
- ½ teaspoon ground cinnamon
- ¼ teaspoon ground ginger (optional, anti-inflammatory)
- Pinch of iodized sea salt
- 1 tablespoon olive oil
- ½ cup fresh or frozen berries

INSTRUCTIONS

1. In a blender or food processor, combine the cooked quinoa, rolled oats, almond milk, beaten egg, flaxseed mixture (if using), cinnamon, ginger (if using), and sea salt. Blend until smooth. The batter may be slightly thick, which is okay.
2. Heat the olive oil in a non-stick skillet over medium heat.
3. Pour about ¼ cup of the batter for each pancake onto the hot skillet.
4. Scatter a few berries on top of each pancake (if using fresh berries). If using frozen berries, gently press them into the batter.
5. Cook for 3-4 minutes per side, or until golden brown and cooked through. You can gently press down on the pancakes with a spatula while cooking to help them cook evenly.
6. Serve warm with additional berries (optional) and a drizzle of maple syrup (use sparingly).

- If the batter seems too thick, add a little more almond milk, one tablespoon at a time, until you reach the desired consistency.
- Leftover pancakes can be stored in an airtight container in the refrigerator for up to 2 days. Gently reheat in a skillet or microwave minutes before serving.
- You can substitute other fruits for the berries like chopped bananas, apples, or peaches.

NUTRITIONAL FACTS

Calories: 150-200

Protein: 4 grams

Fiber: 3 grams

Iron: Good source (from quinoa)

CHAPTER 7

VIBRANT LUNCH OPTIONS

RAINBOW VEGGIE WRAP

Yields: 1 Serving | **Prep Time**: 10 minutes | **Cook Time**: No Cook

INGREDIENTS

- 1 whole wheat tortilla
- ½ cup chopped red bell pepper
- ½ cup chopped orange bell pepper
- ½ cup shredded green cabbage
- ½ cup cooked chickpeas, rinsed and drained
- 2 tablespoons hummus (optional)
- ¼ teaspoon ground cumin (optional, anti-inflammatory)
- Pinch of iodized sea salt
- Lettuce or spinach leaves (optional)

INSTRUCTIONS

1. Wash and chop the bell peppers and cabbage.
2. Warm the whole wheat tortilla in a dry skillet or microwave for a few seconds to make it more pliable (optional).
3. Spread hummus on the tortilla if using.
4. Layer the chopped bell peppers, cabbage, and chickpeas on the tortilla.
5. Season with cumin (if using) and a pinch of sea salt.
6. If using lettuce or spinach leaves, add them for extra texture and nutrients.
7. Roll up the tortilla tightly and enjoy!

- Feel free to add other chopped vegetables to your wrap like shredded carrots, cucumber, or sliced avocado.
- You can substitute the hummus with a light vinaigrette dressing for a lower-fat option.
- Leftover wraps can be stored in an airtight container in the refrigerator for up to 2 days.

NUTRITIONAL FACTS

Calories: 300-350

Protein: 10 grams (from chickpeas)

Fiber: 6 grams

Vitamin C: Excellent source (from bell peppers)

LENTIL SOUP WITH BROWN RICE

Yields: 2-3 servings | **Prep Time:** 15 minutes | **Cook Time:** 30-35 minutes

INGREDIENTS

- 1 cup brown rice, rinsed
- 1½ cups vegetable broth
- 1 cup dried lentils, rinsed
- 2 cups chopped carrots
- 1 cup chopped celery
- 1 onion, chopped
- 2 cloves garlic, minced
- 1 teaspoon dried thyme
- ½ teaspoon ground turmeric
- Pinch of iodized sea salt
- Black pepper to taste
- Olive oil

INSTRUCTIONS

1. In a large pot, heat a drizzle of olive oil over medium heat (optional). Add the chopped onion and cook for 3-4 minutes, or until softened.
2. Add the chopped carrots and celery to the pot and cook for another 5 minutes, or until slightly softened.
3. Stir in the minced garlic, dried thyme, turmeric , and a pinch of sea salt. Cook for another minute until fragrant.
4. Add the rinsed lentils and brown rice to the pot.
5. After adding the veggie broth, bring it to a boil.
6. Reduce heat, cover the pot, and simmer for 30-35 minutes, or until the lentils and rice are cooked through and the liquid is absorbed.
7. Season with black pepper to taste.
8. Serve warm in bowls.

- You can use canned lentils instead of dried lentils to save time. If using canned lentils, add them to the pot with the broth in step 4 and simmer for 10-15 minutes, or until heated through.
- Leftover lentil soup can be stored in an airtight container in the refrigerator for up to 3 days. Reheat on low heat in a saucepan over the stove.

NUTRITIONAL FACTS

Calories: 300-350

Protein: 15 grams (from lentils)

Fiber: 8 grams

Manganese: Excellent source

BLACK BEAN BURGERS

Yields: 2 Burgers | **Prep Time:** 15 minutes | **Cook Time: 10-12 minutes per side**

INGREDIENTS

- 1 can (15 oz) black beans, drained and rinsed
- ½ cup cooked quinoa
- ½ ripe avocado, mashed
- ¼ cup chopped red onion
- 1 tablespoon chopped fresh cilantro
- 1 tablespoon ground cumin
- ½ teaspoon chili powder (optional)
- Pinch of iodized sea salt
- Black pepper to taste
- Cooking spray

INSTRUCTIONS

1. In a large bowl, mash the drained and rinsed black beans with a fork. You can leave some beans slightly chunky for texture.
2. Add the cooked quinoa, mashed avocado, chopped onion, cilantro, cumin, chili powder (if using), sea salt, and black pepper.
3. Mix well to combine all ingredients.
4. Form the mixture into two equal-sized patties.
5. Warm up a grill pan or skillet with a mild oil over a medium-high temperature.
6. Coat the burger patties with cooking spray.
7. Place the patties on the preheated skillet and cook for 5-6 minutes per side, or until golden brown and cooked through. You can also grill the patties for a smoky flavor.
8. Serve the black bean burgers on whole wheat buns with your favorite toppings like lettuce, tomato, sliced onion, and avocado slices.

- If the mixture seems too wet and difficult to form patties, add a tablespoon of bread crumbs or rolled oats to help bind the ingredients.
- You can bake the black bean burgers instead of frying them. Preheat your oven to 400°F (200°C). Place the patties on a baking sheet coated with cooking spray and bake for 15-20 minutes per side, or until cooked through.
- Leftover black bean burgers can be stored in an airtight container in the refrigerator for up to 2 days. Serve warm, straight from the pan or microwave.

NUTRITIONAL FACTS

Calories: 300-350

Protein: 15 grams (from black beans and quinoa)

Fiber: 8 grams

Healthy fats: Good source (from avocado)

SALMON WITH ROASTED VEGETABLES

Yields: 1 Serving | **Prep Time**: 10 minutes | **Cook Time**: 15-20 minutes

INGREDIENTS

- 4 ounces salmon filet
- 1 cup chopped broccoli florets
- ½ cup chopped asparagus spears
- 1 tablespoon olive oil
- ¼ teaspoon dried oregano (optional, anti-inflammatory)
- Pinch of iodized sea salt
- Freshly ground black pepper to taste

INSTRUCTIONS

1. Preheat your oven to 400°F (200°C). Lightly grease a baking sheet.
2. In a bowl, toss the chopped broccoli and asparagus with olive oil, oregano (if using), sea salt, and black pepper.
3. On the baking sheet that has been cleaned, arrange the seasoned vegetables.
4. Place the salmon filet on top of the vegetables.
5. Bake for 15-20 minutes, or until the salmon is cooked through and flakes easily with a fork and the vegetables are tender-crisp.

- You can substitute other vegetables for the broccoli and asparagus such as green beans, Brussels sprouts, or cherry tomatoes.
- Leftover salmon and vegetables can be stored in an airtight container in the refrigerator for up to 2 days.
- Gently reheat in a skillet or microwave shortly before serving.
- For extra flavor, you can marinate the salmon in a mixture of olive oil, lemon juice, and your favorite herbs for 15-30 minutes before baking. Avoid marinades with processed oils like canola or vegetable oil.

NUTRITIONAL FACTS

Calories: 400-450

Protein: 30 grams (from salmon)

Healthy fats: Excellent source (from salmon)

Vitamin C: Good source (from broccoli)

Vitamin A: Good source (from salmon)

TUNA SALAD WITH WHOLE WHEAT CRACKERS

Yields: 1 Serving | **Prep Time:** 10 minutes | **Cook Time:** No Cook

INGREDIENTS

- Five ounces of drained canned tuna (packed in water)
- ½ cup chopped celery
- ¼ cup chopped red onion
- 2 tablespoons plain Greek yogurt
- 1 tablespoon mashed avocado (instead of mayonnaise)
- 1 tablespoon chopped fresh dill (optional)
- Pinch of iodized sea salt
- Freshly ground black pepper to taste
- Whole wheat crackers

INSTRUCTIONS

1. In a bowl, combine the drained tuna, chopped celery, and chopped red onion.
2. Stir in the Greek yogurt, mashed avocado, dill (if using), sea salt, and black pepper.
3. Mix well to combine all ingredients.
4. Serve the tuna salad on whole wheat crackers.

- You can substitute chopped bell pepper, carrots, or cucumbers for the celery.

- If you don't have fresh dill, you can use ¼ teaspoon of dried dill weed.

- Leftover tuna salad can be stored in an airtight container in the refrigerator for up to 2 days. Serve with additional crackers or lettuce leaves.

NUTRITIONAL FACTS

Calories: 300-350

Protein: 25 grams (from tuna)

Healthy fats: Good source (from tuna and avocado)

Vitamin K: Good source (from celery)

CHICKEN AND BROWN RICE SALAD WITH CRANBERRIES

Yields: 1-2 servings | **Prep Time:** 15 minutes | **Cook Time:** Depending on Chicken Cooking Method

INGREDIENTS

- 4 ounces cooked, shredded chicken breast
- ½ cup cooked brown rice
- ¼ cup dried cranberries
- ¼ cup chopped celery
- 2 tablespoons chopped almonds
- 1 tablespoon olive oil
- 2 tablespoons lemon juice
- Pinch of iodized sea salt
- Freshly ground black pepper to taste

INSTRUCTIONS

1. Cook the chicken breast according to your preferred method (baking, grilling, poaching, etc.) until cooked through. Shred the chicken with two forks.
2. In a large bowl, combine the cooked and shredded chicken, cooked brown rice, dried cranberries, chopped celery, and chopped almonds.
3. In a small bowl, whisk together the olive oil, lemon juice, sea salt, and black pepper.
4. Pour the dressing over the chicken and rice mixture and toss to coat evenly.
5. Serve immediately or refrigerate for at least 30 minutes for the flavors to develop.

- Leftover chicken and brown rice salad can be stored in an airtight container in the refrigerator for up to 3 days. Gently reheat in a skillet or microwave shortly before serving.
- You can add a tablespoon of chopped fresh parsley or cilantro for extra flavor and nutrients.
- If you prefer a creamier salad, add a dollop of plain Greek yogurt or mashed avocado to the dressing. Avoid using sour cream or mayonnaise due to their high omega-6 content.

NUTRITIONAL FACTS

Calories: 400-450

Protein: 30 grams (from chicken)

Fiber: 4 grams (from brown rice)

Vitamin C: Good source (from celery)

Manganese: Good source (from brown rice)

SPICY SHRIMP STIR-FRY WITH BOK CHOY AND EDAMAME

Yields: 1 Serving | **Prep Time:** 10 minutes | **Cook Time:** 10-12 minutes

INGREDIENTS

- 4 ounces peeled and deveined shrimp
- 1 cup chopped bok choy (white and green parts)
- ½ cup frozen shelled edamame, thawed
- ½ cup chopped bell pepper (any color)
- 1 tablespoon olive oil
- ½ teaspoon grated ginger
- 1 clove garlic, minced
- Pinch of red pepper flakes (optional, anti-inflammatory)
- Pinch of iodized sea salt
- Freshly ground black pepper to taste

INSTRUCTIONS

1. In a big saucepan or wok over a medium-high temperature, heat the olive oil.
2. Cook the shrimp for two to three minutes on each side, or until they are cooked through and pink.
3. After removing them from the pan, set the shrimp aside.
4. Add the chopped bok choy, bell pepper, and ginger to the pan. Stir-fry for 2-3 minutes, or until the vegetables are slightly softened.
5. Add the edamame and red pepper flakes (if using) to the pan and stir-fry for another minute.
6. Add sea salt and black pepper according to taste.
7. Return the cooked shrimp to the pan and stir-fry for another minute to heat through.
8. Serve immediately over brown rice (optional) or enjoy on its own.

- You can substitute chicken or tofu for the shrimp if preferred.
- Feel free to add other chopped vegetables like broccoli florets, carrots, or snow peas.
- If you don't have fresh ginger, you can use ¼ teaspoon of ground ginger.
- You can keep leftovers in the fridge for up to two days if you store them in an airtight container.
- Gently reheat in a skillet or microwave shortly before serving.

NUTRITIONAL FACTS

Calories: 350-400

Protein: 30 grams (from shrimp)

Healthy fats: Good source (from shrimp)

Vitamin C: Good source (from bok choy)

TOFU LETTUCE WRAPS WITH PEANUT SAUCE

Yields: 2-3 Servings | **Prep Time:** 15 minutes | **Cook Time:** No Cook Time

INGREDIENTS

- 1 block (14 oz) firm tofu, drained and pressed
- 2 tablespoons reduced-sodium soy sauce
- 1 tablespoon rice vinegar
- 1 tablespoon lime juice
- 1 teaspoon grated ginger
- 1 clove garlic, minced
- 1 tablespoon creamy unsalted peanut butter (no added sugar) Limit portion due to peanut content
- 1 tablespoon honey (optional)
- 1 red bell pepper, thinly sliced
- 1 cup shredded carrots
- 1 romaine lettuce heart, leaves separated and washed
- Chopped fresh cilantro (optional)

INSTRUCTIONS

1. For the Peanut Sauce: In a small bowl, whisk together the soy sauce, rice vinegar, lime juice, ginger, garlic, peanut butter, and honey (if using). Set aside.
2. For the Tofu: Cut the tofu into bite-sized cubes. You can pan-fry the tofu cubes in a little olive oil for a few minutes on each side to add a crispy texture (optional).
3. Assemble the Wraps: Place a few tablespoons of peanut sauce on a lettuce leaf. Top with tofu cubes, bell pepper slices, shredded carrots, and chopped cilantro (if using).
4. Fold the bottom of the lettuce leaf up and over the filling, then roll up tightly to create a wrap.
5. Repeat with remaining ingredients.

- You can use ground turkey or chicken breast instead of tofu for a different protein option.

- If you don't have romaine lettuce, you can use butter lettuce leaves or large collard greens.

- The peanut sauce can be stored in an airtight container in the refrigerator for up to a week.

- Leftover tofu cubes can be stored in an airtight container in the refrigerator for up to 3 days. Use them in other recipes like salads or stir-fries.

NUTRITIONAL FACTS

Calories: 300-350

Protein: 20 grams (from tofu)

Healthy fats: Good source (from peanut butter)

Vitamin A: Excellent source (from carrots)

TURKEY AND SWEET POTATO CHILI

Yields: 4-6 servings | **Prep Time:** 15 minutes | **Cook Time:** 30-35 minutes

INGREDIENTS

- 1 pound ground turkey breast
- 1 tablespoon olive oil
- 1 onion, chopped
- 1 green bell pepper, chopped
- 2 cloves garlic, minced
- 1 teaspoon ground cumin
- ½ teaspoon chili powder (optional, anti-inflammatory)
- Pinch of red pepper flakes (optional, anti-inflammatory)
- 1 (15 oz) can diced tomatoes, undrained
- 1 (15 oz) can kidney beans, rinsed and drained
- 1 (15 oz) can black beans, rinsed and drained
- 1 medium sweet potato, peeled and diced
- 4 cups low-sodium chicken broth
- Pinch of iodized sea salt
- Freshly ground black pepper to taste

INSTRUCTIONS

1. Heat the olive oil in a large pot or Dutch oven over medium heat.
2. Add the ground turkey and cook, breaking it up with a spoon, until browned.
3. Add the chopped onion and green pepper to the pot and cook for 5 minutes, or until softened.
4. Stir in the minced garlic, cumin, chili powder (if using), and red pepper flakes (if using). Cook for another minute until fragrant.
5. Add the diced tomatoes (with their juices), kidney beans, black beans, diced sweet potato, and chicken broth to the pot.
6. Bring to a boil, then reduce heat and simmer for 30-35 minutes, or until the sweet potato is tender and the chili has thickened.
7. Add sea salt and black pepper according to taste.

- You can substitute ground chicken or lean ground beef for the ground turkey breast.
- If you like a thicker chili, mash some of the cooked beans against the side of the pot with a fork.
- Remaining food can be frozen for up to three months or kept in the refrigerator for up to three days when kept in an airtight container.
- Reheat gently in a pot on the stovetop before serving.
- Serve the chili with your favorite toppings like chopped avocado, shredded cheese, sour cream (use sparingly), chopped fresh cilantro, or a dollop of plain Greek yogurt.

NUTRITIONAL FACTS

Calories: 400-450

Protein: 30 grams (from turkey and beans)

Fiber: 10 grams (from beans and sweet potato)

Vitamin A: Excellent source (from sweet potato)

MEDITERRANEAN CHICKPEA SALAD SANDWICH

Yields: 1 Serving | **Prep Time:** 10 minutes | **Cook Time:** No Cook

INGREDIENTS

- 1 can (15 oz) chickpeas, rinsed and drained
- 1 roma tomato, diced
- ½ cucumber, diced
- ¼ cup crumbled feta cheese (optional)
- 2 tablespoons chopped Kalamata olives
- 1 tablespoon olive oil
- 1 tablespoon lemon juice
- Pinch of dried oregano
- Pinch of iodized sea salt
- Freshly ground black pepper to taste
- 2 slices whole wheat bread

INSTRUCTIONS

1. In a bowl, combine the chickpeas, diced tomato, diced cucumber, feta cheese (if using), and chopped olives.
2. In a small bowl, whisk together the olive oil, lemon juice, oregano, sea salt, and black pepper.
3. After pouring the dressing over the chickpea mixture, toss to ensure even coating.
4. Toast the whole wheat bread slices (optional).
5. Spread half of the chickpea salad mixture on one slice of bread. Top with the other slice of bread.

TIPS

- You can add other chopped vegetables to the salad like chopped red onion, bell peppers, or celery.
- If you don't have feta cheese, you can omit it or substitute with crumbled low-fat ricotta cheese.
- Leftover chickpea salad can be stored in an airtight container in the refrigerator for up to 3 days. Serve on lettuce leaves or whole wheat crackers for a lighter option.

NUTRITIONAL FACTS

Calories: 350-400

Protein: 15 grams (from chickpeas)

Fiber: 6 grams (from chickpeas)

Healthy fats: Good source (from olive oil)

CHAPTER 8

SATISFYING DINNERS

MANGO SALSA AND SALMON DISH

Yields: **1 Serving** | **Prep Time**: 15 minutes | **Cook Time**: 15-20 minutes

INGREDIENTS

- 4 ounces salmon filet
- 1 ripe mango, diced
- ½ cup chopped tomatoes (any variety)
- ¼ cup chopped red onion
- ¼ cup chopped fresh cilantro
- 1 tablespoon lime juice
- Pinch of iodized sea salt
- Freshly ground black pepper to taste

INSTRUCTIONS

1. Preheat your oven to 400°F (200°C). Lightly grease a baking sheet.
2. In a bowl, combine the diced mango, chopped tomatoes, red onion, and cilantro.
3. Add the lime juice, sea salt, and black pepper to the salsa mixture and toss to coat evenly.
4. After the baking pan is ready, put the salmon filet on it.
5. Place a spoonful of the mango salsa on top of the salmon.
6. Bake for 15-20 minutes, or until the salmon is cooked through and flakes easily with a fork.

- You can substitute other fruits for the mango in the salsa, such as pineapple, peaches, or papaya.
- If you don't have fresh cilantro, you can use 1 tablespoon of chopped fresh parsley.
- Leftover salmon and salsa can be stored in an airtight container in the refrigerator for up to 2 days. Gently reheat in an oven or microwave shortly before serving.

NUTRITIONAL FACTS

Calories: 400-450

Protein: 30 grams (from salmon)

Healthy fats: Excellent source (from salmon)

Vitamin C: Good source (from tomatoes)

Vitamin A: Excellent source (from mango)

TURMERIC CHICKEN WITH ROASTED BRUSSELS SPROUTS

Yields: 1-2 servings | **Prep Time**: 15 minutes | **Cook Time**: 30-35 minutes

INGREDIENTS

- 4 ounces boneless, skinless chicken breast
- 1 tablespoon olive oil
- ½ teaspoon ground turmeric (anti-inflammatory)
- Pinch of iodized sea salt
- Freshly ground black pepper to taste
- 1 cup Brussels sprouts, trimmed and halved
- 2 cloves garlic, minced
- 1 tablespoon chopped fresh parsley (optional)

INSTRUCTIONS

1. Preheat your oven to 400°F (200°C). Lightly grease a baking sheet.
2. In a small bowl, combine the olive oil, turmeric, sea salt, and black pepper.
3. Rub the spice mixture all over the chicken breast.
4. Place the chicken breast on the prepared baking sheet.
5. Toss the halved Brussels sprouts with the minced garlic and a drizzle of olive oil.
6. Place the Brussels sprouts on the baking pan in a circle around the chicken.
7. Bake for 30-35 minutes, or until the chicken is cooked through and the Brussels sprouts are tender-crisp.
8. Garnish with chopped fresh parsley (if using) before serving.

- You can add other vegetables to the baking sheet, such as chopped carrots, broccoli florets, or green beans.
- If you prefer, you can grill the chicken breast instead of baking it.
- Leftover chicken and Brussels sprouts can be stored in an airtight container in the refrigerator for up to 3 days.Gently reheat in an iron skillet or microwave shortly before serving.

NUTRITIONAL FACTS

Calories: 350-400

Protein: 30 grams (from chicken)

Fiber: 4 grams (from Brussels sprouts)

Vitamin C: Excellent source (from Brussels sprouts)

Manganese: Good source (from Brussels sprouts)

HEARTY LENTIL SOUP WITH WHOLE WHEAT BREAD

Yields: 2-3 servings | **Prep Time:** 15 minutes | **Cook Time:** 30-35 minutes

INGREDIENTS

- 1 cup dry lentils, rinsed
- 4 cups low-sodium vegetable broth
- 1 cup chopped carrots
- 1 cup chopped celery
- 1 onion, chopped
- 2 cloves garlic, minced
- 1 teaspoon dried thyme
- Pinch of iodized sea salt
- Freshly ground black pepper to taste
- 2 slices whole wheat bread, toasted (optional)

INSTRUCTIONS

1. In a large pot, combine the rinsed lentils, vegetable broth, chopped carrots, celery, onion, and minced garlic.
2. Bring to a boil, then reduce heat and simmer for 30-35 minutes, or until the lentils are tender and the soup has thickened.
3. Stir in the dried thyme, sea salt, and black pepper to taste.
4. To give the flavors time to blend, boil the soup for a few more minutes.
5. If you prefer a smoother soup, you can use an immersion blender to puree some or all of the soup.
6. Serve the lentil soup hot with a slice or two of toasted whole wheat bread.

- You can add other chopped vegetables to the soup, such as green beans, potatoes, or spinach.
- If you like a heartier soup, you can add a can of diced tomatoes (undrained) or a cooked, shredded chicken breast.
- Leftover lentil soup can be stored in an airtight container in the refrigerator for up to 3 days or frozen for up to 3 months. Reheat gently in a pot on the stovetop before serving.

NUTRITIONAL FACTS

Calories: 300-350

Protein: 15 grams (from lentils)

Fiber: 10 grams (from lentils)

Vitamin A: Good source (from carrots)

TURKEY BURGERS WITH SWEET POTATO FRIES

Yields: 2 servings | **Prep Time:** 15 minutes | **Cook Time:** 15-20 minutes

INGREDIENTS

- 1 pound ground turkey breast
- ½ medium sweet potato, peeled and diced
- ¼ cup chopped onion
- 1 tablespoon olive oil
- ½ teaspoon dried thyme (optional)
- Pinch of iodized sea salt
- Freshly ground black pepper to taste
- 2 whole wheat hamburger buns (optional)

- For the Sweet Potato Fries:
- One medium sweet potato, sliced into wedges after peeling
- 1 tablespoon olive oil
- Pinch of iodized sea salt
- Freshly ground black pepper to taste

INSTRUCTIONS

For the Turkey Burgers:

1. Preheat a grill pan or large skillet over medium heat.
2. In a large bowl, combine the ground turkey, diced sweet potato, chopped onion, thyme (if using), sea salt, and black pepper.
3. Mix well and gently form the mixture into two equal-sized patties.
4. Apply a thin layer of olive oil to the patties.
5. Place the turkey burgers on the preheated grill pan or skillet and cook for 7-8 minutes per side, or until cooked through.

For the Sweet Potato Fries:

1. Preheat your oven to 400°F (200°C). Lightly grease a baking sheet.
2. Toss the sweet potato wedges with olive oil, sea salt, and black pepper.
3. Spread the sweet potato wedges in a single layer on the prepared baking sheet.
4. Bake for 15-20 minutes, or until tender-crisp, flipping halfway through cooking.

Assembly:

- Serve the cooked turkey burgers on whole wheat hamburger buns (if using) with the sweet potato fries on the side.

TIPS

- You can add other chopped vegetables to the turkey burgers, such as mushrooms, zucchini, or bell peppers.
- If you don't have a grill pan, you can cook the turkey burgers in a skillet with a little olive oil.
- Leftover turkey burgers and sweet potato fries can be stored in an airtight container in the refrigerator for up to 3 days. Gently warm up in a skillet or microwave shortly before serving.

NUTRITIONAL FACTS

Calories: 400-450

Protein: 30 grams (from turkey)

Healthy fats: Good source (from olive oil)

Vitamin A: Excellent source (from sweet potato)

RAINBOW VEGGIE FAJITAS

Yields: 2 servings | **Prep Time:** 10 minutes | **Cook Time:** 10-12 minutes

INGREDIENTS

- 1 bell pepper (any color), sliced
- ½ summer squash, sliced
- ½ red onion, sliced
- 1 tablespoon olive oil
- ½ teaspoon ground cumin (optional)
- Pinch of iodized sea salt
- Freshly ground black pepper to taste
- 2 whole wheat tortillas

Optional Toppings:

- Chopped fresh cilantro or parsley
- Sliced avocado
- Low-fat shredded cheese
- Salsa

INSTRUCTIONS

1. On medium-high temperatures, warm the olive oil in a big skillet or saucepan.
2. Add the sliced bell pepper, summer squash, and red onion to the pan.
3. Stir-fry the vegetables for five to seven minutes, or until they are crisp-tender.
4. Stir in the ground cumin (if using), sea salt, and black pepper.
5. Warm the whole wheat tortillas according to package instructions (optional).

Assembly:

6. Fill each tortilla with the stir-fried vegetables.
7. Add your desired toppings, such as chopped fresh cilantro, sliced avocado, low-fat shredded cheese, or salsa.
8. Fold the tortillas in half and enjoy.

- You can use other vegetables in this recipe, such as broccoli florets, mushrooms, or zucchini.

- If you don't have cumin, you can use another anti-inflammatory spice like turmeric or ginger.

- Leftover stir-fried vegetables can be stored in an airtight container in the refrigerator for up to 3 days. Gently reheat in a skillet or microwave shortly before serving.

NUTRITIONAL FACTS

Calories: 300-350

Fiber: Good source (from vegetables and tortillas)

Vitamin C: Good source (from bell peppers)

TOFU STIR-FRY WITH BROCCOLI AND BROWN RICE

Yields: 1 Serving | **Prep Time:** 10 minutes | **Cook Time:** 15-20 minutes

INGREDIENTS

- 1 block (14 oz) firm tofu, drained and pressed
- 1 cup chopped broccoli florets
- ½ cup cooked brown rice
- 1 tablespoon olive oil
- 1 tablespoon grated ginger
- 1 clove garlic, minced
- Pinch of iodized sea salt
- Freshly ground black pepper to taste

INSTRUCTIONS

For the Tofu:

1. Cut the tofu into bite-sized cubes.
2. You can pan-fry the tofu cubes in a little olive oil for a few minutes on each side to add a crispy texture (optional).
3. Heat the remaining olive oil in a large skillet or wok over medium-high heat.
4. Add the chopped broccoli florets and stir-fry for 3-4 minutes, or until tender-crisp.
5. Add the grated ginger and minced garlic to the pan and cook for another minute until fragrant.
6. Add the cooked brown rice and stir-fry for another minute or two to heat through.
7. If you pan-fried the tofu, add it back to the pan with the vegetables and rice.
8. To taste, add black pepper and sea salt for seasoning.

TIPS

- You can add other chopped vegetables to the stir-fry, such as carrots, bell peppers, or snap peas.
- If you don't have fresh ginger, you can use ¼ teaspoon of ground ginger.
- You can keep leftovers in the fridge for up to two days if you store them in an airtight container.
- Gently reheat in a saucepan or microwave shortly before serving.

NUTRITIONAL FACTS

Calories: 400-450

Protein: 20 grams (from tofu)

Fiber: 5 grams (from tofu and brown rice)

Vitamin C: Good source (from broccoli)

SALMON WITH ROASTED ASPARAGUS AND QUINOA

Yields: 1 Serving | **Prep Time:** 15 minutes | **Cook Time:** 20-25 minutes

INGREDIENTS

- 4 ounces salmon filet
- 1 cup chopped asparagus spears
- ½ cup rinsed quinoa
- 1 tablespoon olive oil
- Pinch of iodized sea salt
- Freshly ground black pepper to taste

INSTRUCTIONS

1. Preheat your oven to 400°F (200°C). Lightly grease a baking sheet.
2. In a small pot, combine the rinsed quinoa with 1 cup of water (or low-sodium vegetable broth for added flavor). Bring to a boil, then reduce heat, cover, and simmer for 15 minutes, or until the quinoa is cooked and fluffy.
3. While the quinoa cooks, toss the chopped asparagus with a drizzle of olive oil and a pinch of sea salt.
4. Arrange the asparagus on one half of the prepared baking sheet.
5. Place the salmon filet on the other half of the baking sheet.
6. Season the salmon with a pinch of sea salt and black pepper.
7. Bake for between fifteen and twenty minutes, or until the asparagus is crisp-tender and the salmon is cooked through and flakes readily with a fork.

- You can substitute other vegetables for the asparagus, such as broccoli florets, green beans, or Brussels sprouts.
- Leftover salmon, asparagus, and quinoa can be stored in an airtight container in the refrigerator for up to 2 days. Gently reheat in a saucepan or microwave shortly before serving.

NUTRITIONAL FACTS

Calories: 450-500

Protein: 30 grams (from salmon)

Healthy fats: Excellent source (from salmon)

Fiber: 4 grams (from quinoa)

LENTIL SHEPHERD'S PIE WITH MASHED SWEET POTATOES

Yields: 2-3 servings | **Prep Time:** 20 minutes | **Cook Time:** 30-35 minutes

INGREDIENTS

- 1 cup dry lentils, rinsed
- 2 cups low-sodium vegetable broth
- 1 cup chopped mixed vegetables (carrots, celery, onions)
- 1 clove garlic, minced
- 1 tablespoon olive oil
- ½ teaspoon dried thyme (optional)
- Pinch of iodized sea salt
- Freshly ground black pepper to taste
- 1 medium sweet potato, peeled and cubed

INSTRUCTIONS

1. In a large pot, combine the rinsed lentils, vegetable broth, chopped vegetables, and minced garlic.
2. Bring to a boil, then reduce heat, cover, and simmer for 20-25 minutes, or until the lentils are tender and the vegetables are softened.
3. While the lentils and vegetables cook, place the peeled and cubed sweet potato in a separate pot with enough water to cover. Bring to a boil, then reduce heat and simmer for 10-15 minutes, or until the sweet potato is tender.
4. Once the sweet potato is cooked, drain the water and mash it with a fork or potato masher. You can add a splash of low-sodium vegetable broth for a smoother texture (optional).
5. Season the lentil mixture with dried thyme (if using), sea salt, and black pepper to taste.

Assembly:

1. Preheat your oven to broil.

2. Spoon the lentil mixture into an oven-safe baking dish.

3. Top the lentil mixture with the mashed sweet potatoes.

4. Broil for a few minutes, or until the top of the sweet potatoes is slightly golden brown.

TIPS

- You can add other chopped vegetables to the lentil mixture, such as green beans, peas, or corn.
- Should you be lacking fresh thyme, you may substitute ¼ teaspoon of dried thyme.
- Leftover lentil shepherd's pie can be stored in an airtight container in the refrigerator for up to 3 days or frozen for up to 3 months. Before serving, reheat slightly in your microwave or oven.

NUTRITIONAL FACTS

Calories: 350-400

Protein: 15 grams (from lentils)

Fiber: 10 grams (from lentils and sweet potato)

Vitamin A: Excellent source (from sweet potato)

CHICKEN AND VEGETABLE STIR-FRY WITH BROWN RICE

Yields: 1 Serving | **Prep Time:** 10 minutes | **Cook Time:** 15-20 minutes

INGREDIENTS

- 4 oz of cooked, shredded, without skin., boneless chicken breast
- 1 cup chopped mixed vegetables (broccoli florets, carrots, bell peppers)
- ½ cup cooked brown rice
- 1 tablespoon olive oil
- 1 tablespoon grated ginger
- 1 clove garlic, minced
- Pinch of iodized sea salt
- Freshly ground black pepper to taste

INSTRUCTIONS

1. Cook the Chicken (if not pre-cooked): If you don't have pre-cooked chicken, you can poach or bake the chicken breast before starting the stir-fry.
2. To poach the chicken, place it in a pot with enough water to cover and bring to a boil. Reduce heat and simmer for 10-12 minutes, or until cooked through.
3. To bake the chicken, preheat your oven to 400°F (200°C). Lightly grease a baking sheet, place the chicken breast on the sheet, and bake for 15-20 minutes, or until cooked through. Once cooked, shred the chicken breast with two forks.
4. On medium-high flames, warm the olive oil in a big skillet or wok.
5. Add the chopped vegetables and stir-fry for 3-4 minutes, or until tender-crisp.
6. Add the grated ginger and minced garlic to the pan and cook for another minute until fragrant.
7. Add the cooked and shredded chicken breast to the pan with the vegetables.

8. Stir in the cooked brown rice and heat through for another minute or two.

9. Add sea salt and black pepper according to taste.

TIPS

- You can use other pre-cooked lean protein sources in this recipe, such as grilled fish, tofu, or shrimp.
- If you don't have fresh ginger, you can use ¼ teaspoon of ground ginger.
- You can keep leftovers in the fridge for up to two days if you store them in an airtight container.
- Gently reheat in a saucepan or microwave shortly before serving.

NUTRITIONAL FACTS

Calories: 400-450

Protein: 30 grams (from chicken)

Fiber: 5 grams (from vegetables and brown rice)

Vitamin C: Good source (from vegetables)

VEGETARIAN STUFFED PEPPERS

Yields: 2-3 servings | **Prep Time**: 15 minutes | **Cook Time**: 40-45 minutes

INGREDIENTS

- 2-3 large bell peppers (any color combination)
- ½ cup rinsed quinoa
- 1 cup chopped mixed vegetables (corn, zucchini, tomatoes)
- 1 onion, chopped
- 1 clove garlic, minced
- 1 tablespoon olive oil
- ½ teaspoon ground cumin (anti-inflammatory)
- Pinch of iodized sea salt
- Freshly ground black pepper to taste

INSTRUCTIONS

6. Preheat your oven to 375°F (190°C).

7. In a small pot, combine the rinsed quinoa with 1 cup of water (or low-sodium vegetable broth for added flavor). Bring to a boil, then reduce heat, cover, and simmer for 15 minutes, or until the quinoa is cooked and fluffy.

8. While the quinoa cooks, prepare the bell peppers. Wash the bell peppers and cut off the tops, removing the seeds and membranes.

9. Heat the olive oil in a big skillet over a medium-high temperature.

10. Cook the chopped onion for a couple of minutes until it becomes tender.

11. Add the minced garlic and chopped vegetables to the pan and cook for another 5 minutes, or until the vegetables are slightly softened.

12. Stir in the cooked quinoa, ground cumin, sea salt, and black pepper.

13. Once the quinoa is mixed in, spoon the vegetable mixture into the prepared bell peppers.

14. Place the stuffed peppers upright in a baking dish. You can add a little water to the bottom of the baking dish to prevent burning (optional).

15. Bake for thirty to thirty-five minutes, or until the filling has been cooked through and the bell peppers are soft.

TIPS

- You can use other vegetables in the filling, such as chopped mushrooms, diced carrots, or chopped spinach.
- If you don't have ground cumin, you can use another anti-inflammatory spice like turmeric or ginger.
- Leftover stuffed peppers can be stored in an airtight container in the refrigerator for up to 3 days. Reheat gently in an oven or microwave before serving.

NUTRITIONAL FACTS

Calories: 300-350

Protein: 5 grams (from quinoa)

Fiber: 5 grams (from vegetables and quinoa)

Vitamin C: Good source (from vegetables)

HEARTY CHICKEN STEW WITH VEGETABLES AND BARLEY

Yields: 2-3 servings | **Prep Time:** 15 minutes | **Cook Time:** 45-50 minutes

INGREDIENTS

- One-pound chicken breasts or thighs, deboned and skinless, sliced into small pieces
- ½ cup rinsed barley
- 4 cups low-sodium chicken broth
- 2 cups chopped mixed vegetables (carrots, celery, potatoes)
- 1 onion, chopped
- 2 cloves garlic, minced
- 1 tablespoon olive oil
- ½ teaspoon dried thyme (optional)
- Pinch of iodized sea salt
- Freshly ground black pepper to taste

INSTRUCTIONS

1. In a large pot or Dutch oven, heat the olive oil over medium heat.
2. Cook until the onion becomes tender, a few minutes after adding it chopped.
3. Add the chicken pieces to the pot and cook for 5-7 minutes, or until lightly browned on all sides.
4. Stir in the minced garlic and cook for another minute until fragrant.
5. Add the rinsed barley, chopped vegetables, low-sodium chicken broth, dried thyme (if using), sea salt, and black pepper.

6. Bring to a boil, then reduce heat, cover the pot, and simmer for 30-35 minutes, or until the barley and vegetables are tender and the chicken is cooked through.

7. You can check for doneness by inserting a fork into the thickest part of a chicken piece.

8. Juices should be clear rather than pink.

TIPS

- You can use other vegetables in this recipe, such as green beans, peas, or corn.
- If you don't have dried thyme, you can use another anti-inflammatory spice like turmeric or ginger.
- Leftover chicken stew can be stored in an airtight container in the refrigerator for up to 3 days or frozen for up to 3 months. Reheat gently in a pot on the stovetop before serving.

Additional Notes:

- This recipe excludes red meat, which can worsen inflammation for some people with osteoarthritis.
- Chicken is a lean protein source and a good alternative.
- Be sure to remove the skin from the chicken pieces before cooking to reduce fat content.

NUTRITIONAL FACTS

Calories: 400-450

Protein: 30 grams (from chicken)

Fiber: 5 grams (from barley and vegetables)

Vitamin A: Good source (from carrots)

SHRIMP SCAMPI WITH WHOLE WHEAT PASTA

Yields: 2-3 servings | **Prep Time:** 15 minutes | **Cook Time:** 15-20 minutes

INGREDIENTS

- 1 pound peeled and deveined shrimp (thawed if frozen)
- ½ pound whole wheat pasta (such as penne or spaghetti)
- 2 tablespoons olive oil
- 3 cloves garlic, minced
- 1 cup chopped tomatoes (fresh or canned)
- ½ cup low-sodium chicken broth
- 1 tablespoon chopped fresh parsley (optional)
- Pinch of iodized sea salt
- Pinch of black pepper

INSTRUCTIONS

1. Follow the directions on the package to cook the whole wheat pasta.
2. Drain and set aside.
3. While the pasta cooks, heat the olive oil in a large skillet or pan over medium heat.
4. Add the minced garlic and cook for a minute until fragrant.
5. Add the shrimp to the pan and cook for 3-5 minutes per side, or until pink and opaque.
6. Stir in the chopped tomatoes and low-sodium chicken broth.
7. After bringing to a simmer, cook for five minutes, or until the sauce starts to gradually thicken.
8. Remove the pan from the heat and stir in the cooked whole wheat pasta and chopped parsley (if using).

9. To taste, add a dash of sea salt and black pepper for seasoning.

TIPS

- You can use other vegetables in this recipe, such as chopped mushrooms, zucchini, or spinach.
- If you don't have fresh parsley, you can use ½ teaspoon dried parsley instead.
- Leftover shrimp scampi can be stored in an airtight container in the refrigerator for up to 2 days.

NUTRITIONAL FACTS

Calories: 400-450

Protein: 30 grams (from shrimp)

Fiber: 5 grams (from whole wheat pasta)

Vitamin C: Good source (from tomatoes)

VEGETARIAN CHILI WITH QUINOA AND BLACK BEANS

Yields: 4-6 servings | **Prep Time:** 15 minutes | **Cook Time:** 40-45 minutes

INGREDIENTS

- 1 cup rinsed quinoa
- One fifteen-oz can of rinsed and drained black beans
- One 15-oz can of washed and drained kidney beans
- 1 (28-ounce) can crushed tomatoes (fire-roasted recommended for added flavor)
- 4 cups low-sodium vegetable broth
- 1 onion, chopped
- 2 cloves garlic, minced
- 1 bell pepper (any color), chopped
- 1 teaspoon ground cumin (anti-inflammatory)
- ½ teaspoon dried oregano (optional)
- Pinch of iodized sea salt
- Pinch of black pepper

INSTRUCTIONS

1. In a large pot or Dutch oven, heat a drizzle of olive oil over medium heat (optional).
2. Cook until the onion becomes tender, a few minutes after adding it chopped.
3. Cook for an additional minute or until fragrant after adding the minced garlic.
4. Stir in the rinsed quinoa, black beans, kidney beans, crushed tomatoes, low-sodium vegetable broth, chopped bell pepper, ground cumin, and dried oregano (if using).
5. Bring to a boil, then reduce heat, cover the pot, and simmer for 30-35 minutes, or until the quinoa is cooked and the chili has thickened.
6. Add a dash of sea salt and black pepper, according to taste.

- You can add other vegetables to this chili, such as chopped carrots, corn, or zucchini.

- If you like a spicier chili, you can add a pinch of cayenne pepper.

- Leftover vegetarian chili can be stored in an airtight container in the refrigerator for up to 3 days or frozen for up to 3 months.

NUTRITIONAL FACTS

Calories: 300-350

Protein: 15 grams (from quinoa and beans)

Fiber: 10 grams (from quinoa and beans)

Vitamin C: Good source (from tomatoes)

SPICED CHICKPEA CURRY WITH BROWN RICE

Yields: 2-3 servings | **Prep Time:** 15 minutes | **Cook Time:** 30-35 minutes

INGREDIENTS

- 1 cup rinsed and drained chickpeas
- 1 cup cooked brown rice
- 1 tablespoon olive oil
- 1 onion, chopped
- 2 cloves garlic, minced
- 1 tablespoon curry powder (anti-inflammatory)
- 1 (14.5-ounce) can diced tomatoes, undrained
- 1 cup low-sodium vegetable broth
- ½ cup unsweetened coconut milk (light coconut milk is preferred)
- Pinch of iodized sea salt
- Pinch of black pepper
- Chopped fresh cilantro for garnish (optional)

INSTRUCTIONS

1. In a large pot or Dutch oven, heat the olive oil over medium heat.
2. Cook until the onion becomes tender, a few minutes after adding it chopped.
3. Cook for an additional minute or until fragrant after adding the minced garlic.
4. Stir in the curry powder and cook for an additional minute, allowing the spices to release their aroma.
5. Add the diced tomatoes (with their juices), low-sodium vegetable broth, and unsweetened coconut milk.
6. Bring to a simmer.
7. Stir in the rinsed and drained chickpeas.
8. Cover the pot, reduce heat, and simmer for 15-20 minutes, or until the chickpeas are heated through and the sauce thickens slightly.
9. While the curry simmers, cook the brown rice according to package instructions.
10. Once the chickpeas are heated through, season the curry with a pinch of sea salt and black pepper to taste.
11. Serve the spiced chickpea curry over a bed of cooked brown rice.

12. Garnish with chopped fresh cilantro (optional).

TIPS

- You can adjust the amount of curry powder to your desired level of spice.

- You can add other vegetables to this curry, such as chopped carrots, bell peppers, or broccoli.

- Leftover spiced chickpea curry can be stored in an airtight container in the refrigerator for up to 3 days.

NUTRITIONAL FACTS

Calories: 400-450

Protein: 15 grams (from chickpeas)

Fiber: 8 grams (from chickpeas and brown rice)

Healthy fats: Good source (from coconut milk)

BAKED COD WITH LEMON AND HERBS

Yields: 2 servings | **Prep Time:** 10 minutes | **Cook Time:** 15-20 minutes

INGREDIENTS

- 2 cod filets (around 6 ounces each)
- 1 tablespoon olive oil
- 1 lemon, sliced
- 2 cloves garlic, minced
- ½ teaspoon dried thyme (anti-inflammatory)
- Pinch of iodized sea salt
- Pinch of black pepper

INSTRUCTIONS

1. Preheat your oven to 400°F (200°C). Lightly grease a baking dish.
2. Use paper towels to wipe the cod filets dry.
3. After the baking dish is ready, put the cod filets in it.
4. Drizzle the cod filets with olive oil.
5. Top the cod with lemon slices, minced garlic, dried thyme, sea salt, and black pepper.
6. Bake the cod for 15-20 minutes, or until the fish flakes easily with a fork and is cooked through.

- For a smoother salsa, mash some of the avocado with a fork before combining with other ingredients.
- If the salsa isn't spicy enough, add a few extra sprinkles of chopped jalapeño.
- Serve immediately with plantain chips or your favorite lectin-free crackers.

NUTRITIONAL FACTS

Calories: 300-350

Protein: 30 grams (from cod)

Healthy fats: Good source (from cod)

CHAPTER 9

SMART SNACKING

BERRY YOGURT PARFAIT

Yields: 1 serving | **Prep Time:** 5 minutes | **Cooking Time:** No cooking

INGREDIENTS

- ½ cup plain, low-fat yogurt (Greek yogurt is a good option)
- A quarter-cup of berries, either fresh or frozen (strawberries, raspberries, and blueberries)
- ¼ cup granola (choose a variety low in sugar and with whole grains)

INSTRUCTIONS

1. In a bowl or parfait glass, layer half of the yogurt.
2. Top the yogurt with half of the berries.
3. Sprinkle half of the granola on top of the berries.
4. Layers with the leftover yogurt, granola, and berries as repeated.

- You can use other fruits in this recipe, such as chopped mango, peaches, or pineapple.

- If using frozen berries, let them thaw slightly before layering in the parfait.

- Choose a granola that is low in added sugar and contains whole grains for extra fiber.

- For a creamier texture, you can stir in a tablespoon of honey or maple syrup to the yogurt before layering.

NUTRITIONAL FACTS

Calories: 250-300

Protein: 15 grams (from yogurt)

Fiber: 3 grams (from yogurt, berries, and granola)

Vitamin C: Excellent source (from berries)

BAKED APPLE CHIPS WITH CINNAMON

Yields: about 1 cup | **Prep Time**: 10 minutes | **Cook Time**: 1-2 hours

INGREDIENTS

- 2 large apples (any variety)
- 1 tablespoon lemon juice (optional)
- ½ teaspoon ground cinnamon

INSTRUCTIONS

1. Preheat your oven to the lowest setting (usually around 200°F or 93°C).
2. Line a baking sheet with parchment paper.
3. Wash and dry the apples. Slice the apples very thin (around 1/8 inch thick) using a sharp knife or mandoline slicer.
4. In a large bowl, toss the apple slices with lemon juice (if using) to prevent browning.
5. Place the apple slices in a single layer on the baking sheet that has been preheated.
6. Sprinkle the apple slices with ground cinnamon.
7. Bake the apple chips for 1-2 hours, or until they are dry and crisp but still slightly flexible. You may need to flip the slices halfway through baking for even drying.
8. Allow the apple chips to cool fully before putting them away.

- You can use different types of apples for this recipe, such as Granny Smith, Gala, or Fuji.
- If your oven does not have a low setting, you can crack the oven door slightly while baking to allow moisture to escape.
- Store leftover baked apple chips in an airtight container at room temperature for up to a week.

NUTRITIONAL FACTS

Calories: 100

Fiber: 4 grams (from apples)

Vitamin C: Good source (from apples)

TRAIL MIX WITH NUTS, SEEDS, AND DRIED FRUIT

Yields: 1 cup | **Prep Time:** 5 minutes | **Cooking Time:** No cooking

INGREDIENTS

- ¼ cup unsalted almonds
- ¼ cup walnuts
- ¼ cup sunflower seeds
- ¼ cup dried cranberries

INSTRUCTIONS

1. In a bowl, combine the almonds, walnuts, sunflower seeds, and dried cranberries.

TIPS

- You can customize this trail mix with other ingredients you enjoy, such as cashews, pecans, raisins, or dried cherries.
- Be sure to choose unsalted nuts and dried fruit with no added sugar for a healthier option.
- Store leftover trail mix in an airtight container at room temperature for up to a week.

NUTRITIONAL FACTS

Calories: 400

Protein: 10 grams (from nuts and seeds)

Fiber: 6 grams (from nuts, seeds, and dried fruit)

Healthy fats: Good source (from nuts and seeds)

HUMMUS WITH VEGGIE STICKS

Yields: 2 servings | **Prep Time:** 5 minutes | **Cooking Time:** No cooking

INGREDIENTS

- 1 cup store-bought hummus (choose a variety with no added sugars or unhealthy fats)
- 2 large carrots, cut into sticks
- 2 celery stalks, cut into sticks
- One bell pepper, sliced into strips, any color

INSTRUCTIONS

2. Wash and prepare the vegetables by cutting them into sticks or strips.
3. Arrange the veggie sticks on a plate.
4. Serve the hummus alongside the veggie sticks for dipping.

- You can choose other vegetables for dipping, such as cucumber slices, sugar snap peas, or broccoli florets.
- If you prefer to make your own hummus, there are many healthy recipes available online.
- Look for hummus options with added roasted red peppers or olives for extra flavor and nutrients.

NUTRITIONAL FACTS

Calories: 200-250

Protein: 5 grams (from hummus)

Fiber: 5 grams (from hummus and vegetables)

Healthy fats: Good source (from hummus)

GUACAMOLE WITH WHOLE WHEAT PITA BREAD

Yields: 1 serving | **Prep Time:** 5 minutes | **Cooking Time:** No cooking

INGREDIENTS

- ½ ripe avocado, mashed
- 1 tablespoon lime juice
- 1 tablespoon chopped tomato
- Pinch of iodized sea salt
- 1 whole wheat pita bread, cut into wedges

INSTRUCTIONS

1. In a bowl, use a fork to crush the avocado.
2. Stir in the lime juice, chopped tomato, and a pinch of sea salt.
3. Taste and adjust seasonings as desired.
4. Serve the guacamole with the whole wheat pita bread wedges for scooping.

TIPS

- In a bowl, use a fork to crush the avocado.
- Stir in the lime juice, chopped tomato, and a pinch of sea salt.
- Taste and adjust seasonings as desired.
- Serve the guacamole with the whole wheat pita bread wedges for scooping.

NUTRITIONAL FACTS

Calories: 250-300

Fiber: 3 grams (from avocado and pita bread)

Healthy fats: Good source (from avocado)

Vitamin C: Good source (from tomato)

EDAMAME PODS WITH SEA SALT

Yields: 1 serving | **Prep Time**: 5 minutes | **Cooking Time**: According to package instructions

INGREDIENTS

- 1 cup frozen edamame pods in shells
- Pinch of iodized sea salt

INSTRUCTIONS

1. Follow the cooking instructions on the package of frozen edamame pods. This may involve boiling, steaming, or microwaving.
2. Once cooked, drain the edamame pods and sprinkle with a pinch of sea salt.
3. Allow the edamame to cool slightly before enjoying.

TIPS

- You can buy edamame pods already shelled if you prefer.
- Edamame pods can be enjoyed hot or cold.
- Sprinkle the edamame with a little paprika or cayenne pepper for a touch of spice (optional).

NUTRITIONAL FACTS

Calories: 200

Protein: 15 grams (from edamame)

Fiber: 8 grams (from edamame

HARD-BOILED EGGS WITH WHOLE WHEAT TOAST

Yields: 1 serving | **Prep Time:** 10 minutes | **Cook Time:** 12-14 minutes

INGREDIENTS

- 1 large egg
- 1 slice whole wheat toast

INSTRUCTIONS

1. Place the egg in a small pot and cover it with cold water.
2. On a medium-high flame, bring your water to a boil.
3. Once boiling, remove the pot from the heat, cover it with a lid, and let the egg sit for 12-14 minutes. This will result in a hard-boiled egg with a firm yolk.
4. While the egg cooks, toast your slice of whole wheat bread in a toaster.
5. After 12-14 minutes, remove the egg from the hot water with a spoon and run cold water over it for a few minutes to stop the cooking process.
6. After peeling, cut the egg in half.
7. Enjoy the hard-boiled egg slices on your toasted whole wheat bread.

TIPS

- You can add a sprinkle of iodized sea salt and black pepper to the egg slices for extra flavor.
- If you prefer a softer yolk, cook the egg for 7-8 minutes instead of 12-14 minutes.
- For a more complete breakfast, add a piece of fruit on the side.

NUTRITIONAL FACTS

Calories: 200

Protein: 12 grams (from egg)

Fiber: 2 grams (from whole wheat toast)

GREEK YOGURT WITH CHIA SEEDS AND BERRIES

Yields: 1 serving | **Prep Time:** 5 minutes | **Cook Time:** No cooking

INGREDIENTS

- ½ cup plain Greek yogurt
- 1 tablespoon chia seeds
- ¼ cup fresh or frozen berries (blueberries, raspberries, strawberries)

INSTRUCTIONS

1. In a bowl, combine the plain Greek yogurt, chia seeds, and berries.
2. Stir everything together and enjoy!

TIPS

- You can use other fruits in this recipe, such as chopped mango, peaches, or pineapple.
- If using frozen berries, let them thaw slightly before adding them to the yogurt.
- For a touch of sweetness, drizzle a little honey or maple syrup on top (optional).

NUTRITIONAL FACTS

Calories: 200

Protein: 15 grams (from Greek yogurt)

Fiber: 5 grams (from Greek yogurt, chia seeds, and berries)

Vitamin C: Good source (from berries)

ROASTED CHICKPEAS WITH HERBS

Yields: about 1 cup **Prep Time:** 10 minutes **Cook Time:** 40-45 minutes

INGREDIENTS

- 1 cup dried chickpeas, rinsed and drained
- 1 tablespoon olive oil
- ½ teaspoon dried thyme (anti-inflammatory)
- Pinch of iodized sea salt
- Pinch of black pepper

INSTRUCTIONS

1. Preheat your oven to 400°F (200°C). Line a baking sheet with parchment paper.
2. In a bowl, toss the rinsed and drained chickpeas with olive oil, dried thyme, sea salt, and black pepper.
3. Arrange the chickpeas on the baking sheet that has been preheated in a single layer.
4. Roast the chickpeas for 40-45 minutes, or until they are golden brown and crispy. You may need to stir them occasionally for even roasting.
5. Let the roasted chickpeas cool slightly before enjoying.

- You can add other spices to the chickpeas for different flavor variations, such as paprika, cumin, or garlic powder.
- Roasted chickpeas can be stored in an airtight container at room temperature for up to a week.
- Enjoy roasted chickpeas as a snack on their own, or add them to salads or yogurt bowls for extra protein and crunch.
- **Please note**: This recipe excludes peanut butter due to its omega-6 content. Here's an alternative recipe using a nut butter suitable for osteoarthritis diets:

NUTRITIONAL FACTS

Calories: 200

Protein: 10 grams (from chickpeas)

Fiber: 6 grams (from chickpeas)

ALMOND BUTTER AND FRUIT ROLL-UPS

Yields: 2-3 roll-ups | **Prep Time:** 5 minutes | **Cook Time:** No cooking

INGREDIENTS

- 2 whole wheat tortillas
- 2 tablespoons almond butter
- ½ cup sliced banana or other fruit (apples, strawberries)

INSTRUCTIONS

1. Spread the almond butter evenly on one side of each whole wheat tortilla.
2. Top the almond butter with your chosen fruit slices (banana, apples, or strawberries).
3. Roll up the tortillas tightly, starting from the short end with the filling.
4. Cut the rolled-up tortillas in half or thirds for easier handling.
5. Enjoy your almond butter and fruit roll-ups as a healthy and satisfying snack!

TIPS

- You can use other nut butters suitable for osteoarthritis diets, such as sunflower seed butter or cashew butter, instead of almond butter.
- If the tortillas are stiff, you can warm them slightly in a microwave or oven for a few seconds to make them more pliable for rolling.
- Wrap leftover almond butter and fruit roll-ups in plastic wrap and store them in the refrigerator for up to 2 days.

NUTRITIONAL FACTS

Calories: 200

Protein: 5 grams (from almond butter)

Fiber: 3 grams (from whole wheat tortilla and fruit)

CHAPTER 10

14-DAY OSTEOARTHRITIS MEAL PLAN

Day	Breakfast	Lunch	Dinner	Snack
1	Berry Blast Smoothie	Rainbow Veggie Wrap	Salmon with Mango Salsa	Hummus with Veggie Sticks
2	Tropical Power Bowl	Lentil Soup with Brown Rice	Turmeric Chicken with Roasted Brussels Sprouts	Trail Mix with Nuts, Seeds, & Dried Fruit
3	Spiced Oatmeal with Berries	Black Bean Burgers	Hearty Lentil Soup with Whole Wheat Bread	Greek Yogurt with Chia Seeds and Berries
4	Overnight Oats with Nuts and Seeds	Chicken and Brown Rice Salad with Cranberries	Shrimp Scampi with Whole Wheat Pasta	Hard-boiled Eggs with Whole Wheat Toast
5	Quinoa Pancakes with Berries	Spicy Shrimp Stir-fry with Bok Choy and Edamame	Vegetarian Chili with Quinoa and Black Beans	Edamame Pods with Sea Salt
6	Sweet Potato Pancakes	Tofu Lettuce Wraps with Peanut Sauce	Spiced Chickpea Curry with Brown Rice	Roasted Chickpeas with Herbs
7	Power Greens Smoothie	Tuna Salad with Whole Wheat Crackers	Baked Cod with Lemon and Herbs	Berry Yogurt Parfait
8	**Repeat a favorite recipe from Days 1-7**			
9	Salmon and Avocado Toast	Turkey and Sweet Potato Chili	Rainbow Veggie Fajitas	Guacamole with Whole Wheat Pita Bread

10	Turmeric Tofu Scramble	Mediterranean Chickpea Salad Sandwich	Tofu Stir-fry with Broccoli and Brown Rice	Baked Apple Chips with Cinnamon
11	Cherry Tomato and Spinach Frittata	Repeat favorite lunch	Repeat favorite dinner	Trail Mix with Nuts, Seeds, & Dried Fruit
12	Repeat favorite breakfast	Repeat favorite lunch	Lentil Shepherd's Pie with Mashed Sweet Potatoes	Hummus with Veggie Sticks
13	Repeat favorite breakfast	Chicken and Vegetable Stir-fry with Brown Rice	Vegetarian Stuffed Peppers	Greek Yogurt with Chia Seeds and Berries
14	Repeat favorite breakfast	Repeat favorite lunch	Hearty Beef Stew with Vegetables and Barley	Fruit and Nut Butter Roll-Ups

5 Home Remedies for Relieving Inflammation Pain

Inflammation is the body's natural response to injury or infection. While it's a helpful process for healing, chronic inflammation can cause pain and discomfort.

Here are 5 safe and easy home remedies to help relieve inflammation pain:

1. Apply Cold Therapy:

What you'll need: Ice pack, wrapped towel

Instructions:

Wrap an ice pack in a thin towel to prevent skin irritation.

Apply the ice pack to the inflamed area for 15-20 minutes at a time.

Repeat every 2-3 hours as needed.

How it works: Cold therapy numbs the area, reducing pain and inflammation. It also helps constrict blood vessels, minimizing swelling.

2. Apply Heat Therapy:

What you'll need: Heating pad, warm compress (rice sock)

Instructions:

Apply a heating pad or warm compress to the inflamed area for 15-20 minutes at a time.

Repeat every 2-3 hours as needed.

How it works: Heat therapy relaxes muscles, improves blood flow, and promotes healing. It can also ease stiffness and discomfort associated with inflammation.

3. Use Anti-Inflammatory Spices:

What you'll need: Turmeric (fresh or ground), ginger (fresh or ground)

Instructions:

You can add a teaspoon of ground turmeric or ginger to warm water or milk (must be plant based milk like almond milk) to make a soothing drink.

Consider incorporating these spices into your cooking for added flavor and anti-inflammatory benefits.

How it works: Turmeric contains curcumin, a powerful anti-inflammatory compound. Ginger also has anti-inflammatory properties that can help reduce pain and swelling.

4. Rest and Elevate:

Instructions:

When experiencing inflammation pain, especially in the legs or feet, try to rest and elevate the affected area above your heart. This helps reduce swelling and promotes drainage of fluids.

How it works: Elevation helps reduce pressure and fluid buildup in the inflamed area, promoting healing and pain relief.

5. Epsom Salt Bath:

What you'll need: Epsom salt (magnesium sulfate)

Instructions:

Fill a warm bath with one to two cups of Epsom salts.

Soak for 20-30 minutes, allowing the magnesium to relax muscles and reduce inflammation.

How it works: Epsom salt is a magnesium sulfate compound. Magnesium helps relax muscles and may reduce pain and inflammation.

CONCLUSION

Congratulations! You've reached the end of your journey through the world of osteoarthritis-friendly recipes.

 By incorporating these delicious and nutritious dishes into your diet, you've taken a significant step towards managing your joint health and reclaiming your active lifestyle.

Remember, food is powerful medicine, and with mindful choices, you can empower your body to move with greater ease and enjoy the activities you love.

This journey doesn't end here. As you continue to explore new recipes and discover the joys of healthy eating, you'll find a renewed sense of well-being and a body that feels ready to take on the day.

Keep experimenting with flavors, textures, and ingredients – there's a whole world of delicious possibilities waiting to be discovered!

We hope this cookbook has been a valuable resource on your path to managing osteoarthritis. We'd love to hear your feedback!

Please take a moment to leave a review on the book, sharing your experience and favorite recipes. Your insights help us continue creating resources that empower seniors to live a vibrant and active life.

So, with a renewed commitment to healthy eating and a heart full of optimism, step forward with confidence and embrace the possibilities that lie ahead.

Remember, a healthy body leads to a happy life, and you are in control!